Cerebrovascular Disease

What Do I Do Now?

SERIES CO-EDITORS-IN-CHIEF

Lawrence C. Newman, MD
Director of the Headache Institute
Department of Neurology
St. Luke's-Roosevelt Hospital Center
New York, New York

Morris Levin, MD
Co-director of the Dartmouth Headache Center
Director of the Dartmouth Neurology Residency Training Program
Section of Neurology
Dartmouth Hitchcock Medical Center
Lebanon, New Hampshire

OTHER VOLUMES IN THE SERIES

Cerebrovascular Disease

SECOND EDITION

Ji Y. Chong, MD
Assistant Professor of Neurology
Weill Cornell Medical College
Chief of Neurology and Director of the Stroke Center
New York-Presbyterian Lower Manhattan Hospital
New York, New York

Michael P. Lerario, MD
Assistant Professor of Clinical Neurology
Weill Cornell Medical College
Attending Physician
New York-Presbyterian Queens Hospital
Flushing, New York

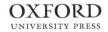
OXFORD
UNIVERSITY PRESS

OXFORD
UNIVERSITY PRESS

Oxford University Press is a department of the University of Oxford. It furthers
the University's objective of excellence in research, scholarship, and education
by publishing worldwide. Oxford is a registered trade mark of Oxford University
Press in the UK and certain other countries.

Published in the United States of America by Oxford University Press
198 Madison Avenue, New York, NY 10016, United States of America.

First Edition published in 2013
Second Edition published in 2017

Library of Congress Cataloging-in-Publication Data
Names: Chong, Ji Y., author. | Lerario, Michael P., author.
Title: Cerebrovascular disease / Ji Y. Chong, Michael P. Lerario.
Description: Second edition. | Oxford ; New York : Oxford University Press,
[2017] | Series: What do I do now? | Includes bibliographical references
and index. | Description based on print version record and CIP data
provided by publisher; resource not viewed.
Identifiers: LCCN 2016018874 (print) | LCCN 2016017898 (ebook) |
ISBN 9780190495558 (e-book) | ISBN 9780190495565 (e-book) |
ISBN 9780190495572 (online) | ISBN 9780190495541 (alk. paper)
Subjects: | MESH: Stroke—diagnosis | Stroke—therapy | Cerebrovascular
Disorders—diagnosis | Cerebrovascular Disorders—therapy | Case Reports
Classification: LCC RC388.5 (print) | LCC RC388.5 (ebook) | NLM WL 356 |
DDC 616.8/1—dc23
LC record available at https://lccn.loc.gov/2016018874

9 8 7 6 5 4 3 2 1
Printed by Webcom, Inc., Canada

Preface

Nearly 800,000 people have a stroke each year in the United States. On average, this means someone has a stroke every 40 seconds. Stroke is the leading cause of disability in the United States and the fifth leading cause of death. These numbers add up to a huge public health problem that needs to be dealt with from all directions: prevention of first and recurrent strokes, diagnosis and acute treatment of stroke, and improving the recovery from stroke.

Neurologists, and specifically vascular neurologists, are the specialists who primarily treat patients with cerebrovascular disease. However, the sheer number of patients with stroke, as well as the multiple risk factors for stroke, guarantees that physicians of all disciplines will see a stroke patient.

Although several unusual cases are presented, most of this book deals with common, practical questions clinicians will encounter. Case presentations highlight evidence-based practice. There are clinical trial data to support many recommendations, but there are also areas in cerebrovascular disease treatment that are still uncertain. Usual practice in the absence of strong data is noted as such.

Cerebrovascular disease is an exciting and evolving field. Since the previous edition, there have been major advancements in acute stroke care through the use of endovascular techniques. Multiple recent clinical trials have demonstrated intra-arterial thrombectomy to be superior to intravenous tissue plasminogen activator alone for some patients with acute intracranial occlusions. As a result, large-scale changes in the systems and coordination of care need to be implemented in order to provide this treatment option to as many eligible patients as possible. Many other novel acute therapies, preventative strategies, and rehabilitation techniques are being investigated, and there is much promise for continued advances in the coming years.

Contents

1 Treatment of Acute Right-Sided Weakness

A 58-year-old woman with hypertension and diabetes presents to the emergency room with right hemiparesis. She had worked her usual night shift and went home and fell asleep at 3:30 a.m. She awoke at 5:30 a.m. and noticed right-sided weakness. She called emergency medical services and arrived at the emergency room at 6:20 a.m. She has a blood pressure of 153/92. She has normal speech and is without any evidence of aphasia. She has a right facial droop. She has prominent weakness of the right arm and leg. Her head computed tomography (CT) scan shows no evidence of hemorrhage or infarct (Fig. 1.1). Her international normalized ratio (INR) and platelet count are normal. It is now 7 a.m.

What do you do now?

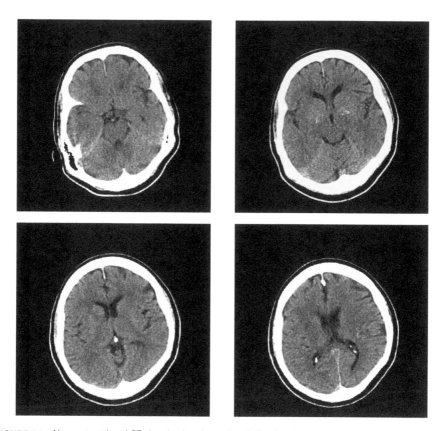

FIGURE 1.1 Noncontrast head CT showing basal ganglia calcifications but otherwise normal findings.

INTRAVENOUS TISSUE PLASMINOGEN ACTIVATOR (IV TPA) FOR ACUTE ISCHEMIC STROKE: INDICATIONS, BENEFITS, AND COMPLICATIONS

This woman is having an acute ischemic stroke. Her symptoms are suggestive of ischemia to the left hemisphere, but there is no language involvement so a large artery occlusion is less likely. A pure motor syndrome involving the face, arm, and leg indicates a small deep infarct. She was last known normal at 3:30 a.m., and we are faced with a decision regarding acute treatment at 7:00 a.m., which is 3.5 hours from onset (onset time is defined as "witnessed onset" or "last known well" in patients with unwitnessed onset—for instance, during sleep).

The benefits of IV tPA have been well established in patients with ischemic stroke treated within 3 hours of symptom onset. The National Institute of Neurological Disorders and Stroke (NINDS) trial of IV tPA administered within 3 hours of acute ischemic stroke showed that there is a significant improvement in outcome compared with placebo. In the NINDS trial, 35% of patients who received placebo recovered to complete independence at 3 months compared to 50% with IV tPA. The inclusion and exclusion criteria for this trial form the basis for the inclusion and exclusion criteria for clinical use of tPA (Box 1.1). Careful patient selection for IV thrombolysis will maximize the benefit and minimize the hemorrhagic risk of treatment. IV tPA remains the mainstay of treatment for acute ischemic stroke, despite recent advances in endovascular therapy for strokes due to large vessel occlusions.

Unfortunately, the rates of tPA use are very low, and one of the major reasons is delay in presentation to the emergency room. Therefore, there has been increased interest in trying to extend the time window for treatment. A pooled analysis of thrombolysis clinical trial data suggested benefit of IV tPA out to 4.5 hours. This led to the European Cooperative Acute Stroke Study (ECASS)

BOX 1.1 **Inclusion/Exclusion Criteria for IV tPA Within 3 Hours of Stroke Onset**

Inclusion

Age >18 years
Clinical diagnosis of ischemic stroke with measurable deficit
Treatment can be initiated within 3 hours

Exclusion

Hemorrhage on head CT
Hypodensity greater than one-third of a cerebral hemisphere on head CT
History of ICH
Subarachnoid hemorrhage
Intracranial neoplasm, arteriovenous malformation, or aneurysm
Minor or rapidly improving symptoms
Seizure at onset with postictal residual impairments
Stroke or head trauma within 3 months
Major surgery within 14 days
Recent intracranial or intraspinal surgery
Acute myocardial infarction within 3 months
Gastrointestinal or genitourinary bleeding within 21 days
Arterial puncture at noncompressible site within 7 days
Heparin within 48 hours and increased partial thromboplastin time
Current use of novel oral anticoagulant within 48 hours or if activated
    partial thromboplastin time or INR remains elevated
INR >1.7 or prothrombin time >15
Platelets <100,000
Aggressive treatment to lower blood pressure <185/110
Glucose <50 or >400

3 trial. In this study, patients in the 3- to 4.5-hour window were randomized to IV tPA 0.9 mg/kg (standard dose) versus placebo. There were additional exclusion criteria beyond those from the NINDS trial: age greater than 80 years, any anticoagulant use (even with INR <1.7), National Institutes of Health Stroke Scale (NIHSS) >25, and history of both prior stroke and diabetes. In the ECASS 3 trial, 45% recovered with placebo and 52% with tPA in the extended window, thus showing a benefit even out to 4.5 hours. Nevertheless, it is well known that the net clinical benefit of IV tPA is optimized the earlier the treatment is initiated.

The major concern with IV tPA is brain hemorrhage risk. In the NINDS trial, 6.8% of the patients treated with IV tPA suffered symptomatic intracerebral hemorrhage (ICH) compared to 0.6% of the patients treated with placebo, with similar mortality between groups. In ECASS 3, the symptomatic ICH rate was higher in the tPA group than in the placebo arm but was comparable to rates

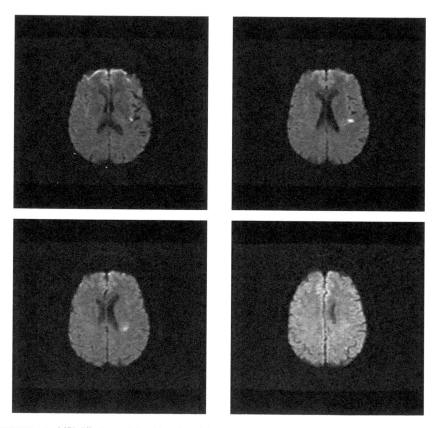

FIGURE 1.2 MRI diffusion-weighted imaging of the brain showing small scattered infarcts in the left hemisphere.

in patients treated within 3 hours. Overall, tPA appears beneficial and without significant additional risk of ICH out to 4.5 hours. Although not US Food and Drug Administration (FDA)-approved in the extended time window, the American Heart Association and other societies have recommended TPA use out to 4.5 hours from stroke onset in select patients.

Post tPA, blood pressure (BP) must be monitored and treated carefully, with a goal BP <180/105. Antihypertensive medications with short duration of action and that are easily titratable are preferred, such as labetalol and nicardipine. For 24 hours following IV thrombolysis, patients cannot receive any antiplatelet or anticoagulant medications and invasive procedures must be avoided.

In this patient, IV tPA was given at 7:20 a.m. (3 hours and 50 minutes after last known well) because she met ECASS 3 criteria for the extended window (i.e., age <80 years, NIHSS <25, no history of diabetes and prior stroke, and no use of anticoagulation). The next day, she had only a slight right arm drift. Her follow-up imaging showed no evidence of hemorrhage and small infarcts on magnetic resonance imaging (MRI) (Fig. 1.2). She was discharged home after 2 days in the hospital.

KEY POINTS TO REMEMBER

· IV tPA is the mainstay of acute ischemic stroke treatment and is FDA-approved within 3 hours of symptom onset.
· Patients benefit when treated early, but the window for treatment may be extended to 4.5 hours in select patients.
· Inclusion and exclusion criteria need to be reviewed carefully to minimize hemorrhage risk and maximize the clinical benefit of tPA.
· Blood pressure monitoring and control is important before and after thrombolysis.

Further Reading

Demaerschalk BM, Kleindorfer DO, Adeoye OM, et al. Scientific rationale for the inclusion and exclusion criteria for intravenous alteplase in acute ischemic stroke: A statement for healthcare professionals from the American Heart Association/American Stroke Association. *Stroke* 2016;47(2):581–641.

Emberson J, Lees KR, Lyden P, et al. Effect of treatment delay, age, and stroke severity on the effects of intravenous thrombolysis with alteplase for acute ischaemic stroke: A meta-analysis of individual patient data from randomised trials. *Lancet* 2014;384(9958):1929–1935.

Hacke W, Kaste M, Bluhmki E, et al. Thrombolysis with alteplase 3 to 4.5 hours after acute ischemic stroke. *N Engl J Med* 2008;359:1317–1329.

Jauch EC, Saver JL, Adams HP Jr, et al. Guidelines for the early management of patients with acute ischemic stroke: A guideline for healthcare professionals from the American Heart Association/American Stroke Association. *Stroke* 2013;44(3):870–947.

The National Institute of Neurological Disorders and Stroke rt-PA Stroke Study Group. Tissue plasminogen activator for acute ischemic. *N Engl J Med* 1995;333(24):1581–1587.

2 Large Vessel Occlusion

An 80-year-old woman with hypertension and atrial fibrillation was admitted to the hospital following a left ankle fracture. Her warfarin was held prior to surgical treatment with internal fixation. Three days after her surgery, she develops acute-onset left-sided weakness and numbness. She also has a right gaze preference and left-sided visual field cut on examination. Her NIHSS is 20, suggesting a high likelihood of a proximal arterial occlusion. Her INR is subtherapeutic since anticoagulation had been held. Her head CT shows only an old right basal ganglia infarct. Her "last seen normal" was 4.5 hours prior during her last vital sign check.

What do you do now?

ENDOVASCULAR TREATMENT FOR ACUTE ISCHEMIC STROKE

This case illustrates some of the limitations of intravenous thrombolysis in acute ischemic stroke. This patient is suspected to be having a severe stroke but is unable to receive IV tPA because she meets two exclusionary criteria: She has had recent major surgery and is outside of the 4.5-hour treatment window. Regardless, this patient likely has a proximal artery occluded given the severity of her symptoms (i.e., her NIHSS score is >10) and the presence of cortical signs (e.g., neglect, aphasia, visual field cut, and gaze preference). In strokes due to proximal arterial occlusions, IV tPA only recanalizes the affected vessel less than one-third of the time. Therefore, this patient should be considered for an alternative acute treatment, such as mechanical clot retrieval, because she is still within a 6-hour treatment window. Mechanical thrombectomy has been shown to have higher rates of recanalization than IV tPA alone and can be used in situations in which tPA may be contraindicated (e.g., recent surgery, coagulation abnormalities, and history of intracranial hemorrhage) because clot extraction does not expose the patient to the systemic effects of pharmacological thrombolysis.

If this patient is not currently at a hospital with capability for neurovascular intervention, she should be immediately transferred to a stroke center that could more thoroughly evaluate whether she meets selection criteria for clot extraction (Box 2.1). At such a center, this patient should be taken emergently for CT angiography in order to confirm that she indeed has a demonstrable proximal artery occlusion (e.g., an occluded internal carotid artery or proximal middle cerebral artery). Two previous studies published in 2013 (SYNTHESIS Expansion and IMS III), which did not evaluate for a proximal arterial occlusion prior to randomization, found no benefit of intra-arterial therapy. In addition, these two trials, along with one other called MR RESCUE, mainly used older generation devices and intra-arterial tPA. Such older methods of treatment have lower rates of recanalization compared to more modern stent retrievers that are used today.

BOX 2.1 **Suggested Emergency Diagnostic Evaluation for Patients with Large Vessel Occlusion**

1. Noncontrast head CT
2. Administer IV tPA if eligible (within 4.5 hours of symptom onset)
3. CT angiography of the head and neck
4. Perform intra-arterial therapy if eligible (within 6 hours for anterior circulation; within 12 hours for posterior circulation)

This and other methadologic issues are the main reasons why these three trials had neutral results.

Two stent retriever devices are currently on the market—Trevo and Solitaire. Both have been used in recent trials demonstrating the benefit of mechanical clot retrieval in acute stroke patients with proximal occlusions. The first and largest of these studies to be published was MR CLEAN. MR CLEAN enrolled 500 acute stroke patients in the Netherlands to compare intra-arterial therapy using a stent retriever with the standard of care, including IV tPA. The authors found that patients receiving treatment with a stent retriever had a 59% chance of arterial recanalization and a 13.5% absolute increase in being functionally independent at 90 days. In response to the publication of Multicenter Randomized Clinical Trial of Endovascular Treatment for Acute Ischemic Stroke in the Netherlands (MR CLEAN), four other enrolling endovascular treatment trials underwent interim analyses and also demonstrated benefit of intervention. These trials included the Endovascular Treatment for Small Core and Anterior Circulation Proximal Occlusion with Emphasis on Minimizing CT to Recenalization Times (ESCAPE), Extending the Time for Thrombolysis in Emergency Neurological Deficits—Intra-Arterial (EXTEND-IA), Solitaire with the Intention for Thrombectomy as Primary Endovascular Treatment for Acute Ischemic Stroke (SWIFT PRIME), and Randomized Trial of Revascularization with Solitaire FR Device Versus Best Medical Therapy (REVASCAT), all published in 2015 (Table 2.1). A meta-analysis of all these trials showed that patients undergoing thrombectomy had a significantly higher rate of angiographic revascularization and improved functional outcomes while having no increase in symptomatic intracranial hemorrhage or mortality. The benefit of endovascular intervention is quite profound: The number needed to treat to obtain one more patient with functional independence ranged from 3 to 4 in these trials. However, the net clinical benefit of treatment diminishes with time, so intra-arterial therapy needs to be initiated as soon as safely possible. In the MR CLEAN trial, for every hour of treatment delay, its absolute benefit was reduced by 6%.

It is important to note that in all the stent retriever trials, the majority of patients undergoing endovascular treatment also were treated with IV tPA. Therefore, patients who are eligible candidates for intravenous thrombolysis should still receive IV tPA within previously defined time windows, as a bridging therapy, while the clinician considers if the patients should be selected for intra-arterial therapy. This is a Class I, Level A recommendation in the most recent guidelines from the American Heart Association.

Our patient was not a candidate for IV tPA; however, she was taken for an emergent CT angiogram, which confirmed an occlusion of the right internal

TABLE 2.1 **Comparison of 2015 Randomized Endovascular Trials**

Trial	N	Age, Mean (Years)[a]	NIHSS, Mean[a]	IV tPA (%)	LKN to Puncture[b]	Successful Recanalization (%)[c]	90-Day Functional Independence (%)[d]		ICH (%)		Mortality (%)	
							IAT	MED	IAT	MED	IAT	MED
MR CLEAN	500	66	17	90	260	59	33	19	7.7	6.4	21	22
ESCAPE	315	71	16	76	200	72	53	29	3.6	2.7	10	19
EXTEND-IA	70	69	17	100	210	86	71	40	0	6	9	20
SWIFT PRIME	196	65	17	98	224	88	60	36	0	3	9	12
REVASCAT	206	66	17	73	269	66	44	28	1.9	1.9	18	16

[a] For IAT arm only. No significant differences reported between control and intervention arms.
[b] Time from last known normal to groin puncture (initiation of procedure) in minutes.
[c] Patients who achieved thrombolysis in cerebral infarction (TICI) 2B/3 (complete or near-complete) revascularization.
[d] Patients who scored 0–2 on the modified Rankin scale at 90 days.

IAT, intra-arterial therapy; ICH, intracerebral hemorrhage; MED, control arm.

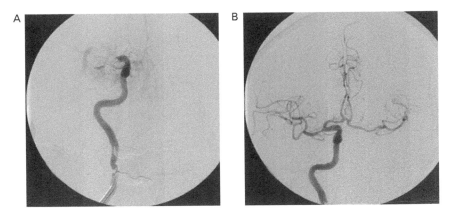

FIGURE 2.1 Cerebral angiogram showing an occluded internal carotid artery terminus (A), followed by complete reperfusion after successful clot removal using a stent retriever (B).

carotid artery terminus. Given that the noncontrast head CT did not show obvious signs of a sizable, completed acute infarct, she was taken for clot extraction with a stent retriever. The interventionalist was able to successfully remove the thrombus and restore full cerebral perfusion (Figure 2.1). The patient immediately improved to her baseline function following the procedure, and the MRI of the brain 1 day later showed only a small completed infarct in the basal ganglia (Figure 2.2).

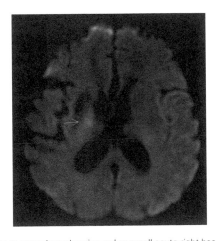

FIGURE 2.2 MRI brain 1 day post-procedure showing only a small acute right basal ganglia infarct.

· Patients eligible for intravenous thrombolysis should receive IV tPA, even if they will later undergo mechanical thrombectomy. However, if ineligible for intravenous thrombolysis, certain patients may still meet selection criteria for intra-arterial treatment.

· A CT angiogram should be used to confirm a proximal arterial occlusion prior to intervention.

· Intra-arterial clot extraction using stent retriever devices has been shown to improve arterial recanalization and functional outcomes in stroke patients with large vessel occlusions. Such procedures should be performed within 6 hours of symptom onset. The sooner treatment is initiated, the better the outcomes.

· If a patient is suffering an ischemic stroke due to a suspected proximal artery occlusion (based on the NIHSS score and the presence of cortical signs), he or she should be transferred to a stroke center capable of performing intra-arterial therapy, if not already at one.

Further Reading

Badhiwala JH, Nassiri F, Alhazzani W. Endovascular thrombectomy for acute ischemic stroke: A meta-analysis. *JAMA* 2015;314(17):1832–1843.

Berkhemer OA, Fransen PS, Beumer D, et al. A randomized trial of intraarterial treatment for acute ischemic stroke. *N Engl J Med* 2015;373(1):11–20.

Fransen PS, Berkhemer OA, Lingsma HF, et al. Time to reperfusion and treatment effect for acute ischemic stroke: A randomized clinical trial. *JAMA Neurol* 2016;73(2):190–196.

Powers WJ, Derdeyn CP, Biller J, et al. 2015 American Heart Association/American Stroke Association focused update of the 2013 guidelines for the early management of patients with acute ischemic stroke regarding endovascular treatment. *Stroke* 2015;46:3024–3039.

3 Masquerade

A 41-year-old woman with hypertension and migraines
presented with acute left arm weakness and numbness
and headache. She had migraines for 5 years with
holocephalic headaches but no aura. Three years prior to
presentation, she was hospitalized at another hospital for
left-sided sensory loss and dysarthria in the setting of a
migraine. She was told she had a stroke. She returned to
normal after that event. The day of this presentation, she
noticed acute left arm weakness and numbness without
involvement of the face or leg. On examination, her blood
pressure was initially 190/105 and spontaneously dropped
to 151/98. She was very uncomfortable from severe
headache. She had a flaccid plegic left arm with anesthesia
of the left arm. She was within the window for IV tPA and
had no contraindications for thrombolysis.

What do you do now?

STROKE MIMIC AND ACUTE TREATMENT

Migraine may be a stroke mimic and, in rare cases, can cause ischemic stroke. In the acute setting, there is little time to complete a full evaluation and wait for resolution of symptoms if tPA is being considered. Therefore, risks and benefits need to be carefully reviewed and discussed with the patient. Hemorrhage rates from tPA increase with higher NIHSS scores since patients with larger strokes are more likely to bleed with tPA. Conversely, patients with stroke mimics are unlikely to have spontaneous ICH because there is no brain infarct.

In one series of 512 patients treated with IV tPA, 14% were thought to have a stroke mimic. The most common diagnoses for these patients were seizure, migraine, and conversion disorder. None had hemorrhagic complications with tPA. Other cohorts of stroke mimic patients also showed low risk of symptomatic ICH following thrombolysis, with the risk estimated to be 1%.

This patient had a history of migraine, and she developed a focal motor deficit in the setting of a migraine attack. On the one hand, her young age and history of migraine make complicated migraine a possibility. However, she had reported a prior history of stroke. She also had hypertension. These factors would increase the risk of recurrent stroke. Furthermore, she had never had motor deficit with migraine before. Therefore, waiting to see if symptoms improve to make a diagnosis of migraine would remove the possibility of treatment if this were indeed stroke. Hospital protocols that employ MRI in the evaluation of acute stroke may help to distinguish stroke mimics from true stroke more accurately than clinical examination and history.

The benefits outweighed the risks of treatment for this patient, and she was given IV tPA. Her symptoms persisted for 3 days, then resolved. Her MRI was subsequently normal and showed no evidence of recent stroke.

This patient was given the diagnosis of complicated migraine and treated with migraine prophylaxis after a complete workup.

KEY POINTS TO REMEMBER

· Patients with stroke mimics likely have a low risk for ICH.
· The benefits outweigh the risks of treatment because the diagnosis of a stroke mimic typically occurs after the tPA window closes.

Further Reading

Chernyshev OY, Martin-Schild S, Albright KC, et al. Safety of tPA in stroke mimics and neuroimaging-negative cerebral ischemia. *Neurology* 2010;74:1340–1345.
Zinkstok SM, Engelter ST, Gensicke H, et al. Safety of thrombolysis in stroke mimics: Results from a multicenter cohort study. *Stroke* 2013;44(4):1080–1084.

4 Improving Symptoms

A 57-year-old man with hypertension and high cholesterol
presented to the emergency room (ER) with acute right
arm weakness and right face numbness. He had no
language or speech involvement. While in the ER, his
symptoms improved, but he was still left with distal hand
weakness and clumsiness. He had no pronator drift and
only slight widening of the right palpebral fissure. His
brain CT was normal.

What do you do now?

MINOR STROKE SYMPTOMS AND ACUTE TREATMENT

More than 30% of patients presenting to medical attention with acute ischemic stroke are found on evaluation to have suffered only minor or rapidly improving deficits. However, minor or rapidly improving stroke symptoms remain a major reason (in one-third of cases) why clinicians exclude patients from receiving intravenous thrombolysis who would otherwise meet criteria for treatment with IV tPA. In the National Institute of Neurological Disorders and Stroke (NINDS) trial, patients were excluded from the study with the following minor symptoms: pure sensory syndrome, isolated dysarthria, isolated facial weakness, and isolated monoparesis with only minor weakness. Minor stroke has been more standardly defined by an NIHSS score of less than 6 in recent trials.

Because these patients were either excluded or underrepresented in the initial landmark trials, one of the contraindications for tPA has historically been mild or rapidly improving symptoms. However, emerging data have demonstrated the relative safety of intravenous thrombolysis in minor stroke patients and a natural history that is not always benign if these patients are left untreated. One study of 29,200 stroke patients who were not treated with IV tPA solely because of rapid improvement or minor symptoms found that 28.3% of these patients were discharged to a facility and 28.5% were dependent for ambulation. Furthermore, the same authors also reported that patients who had more than a 4-point improvement on the NIHSS were more likely to have subsequent worsening. This is consistent with clinical observation that rapid improvement is often a more ominous sign than static symptoms. Rapid improvement implies a dynamic state and is often followed by worsening. If worsening occurs outside the IV tPA window, the patient has lost his or her opportunity for treatment. In addition, hemorrhage risk following thrombolysis has been shown to increase with increasing stroke severity. For example, in the NINDS trial, rates of intracerebral hemorrhage following treatment with IV tPA ranged from 2% (if NIHSS was <6) to 17% (if NIHSS was >20). A total of 5910 minor stroke patients were recently analyzed for rates of adverse events in the Get with the Guidelines–Stroke Registry. This study demonstrated a low risk of hemorrhage (1.8%) and mortality (1.3%) following thrombolysis of minor stroke. Although no randomized trials have rigorously evaluated the use of IV tPA in patients with minor stroke syndromes, it appears that the usage of thrombolytics in these patients should be safe from a hemorrhage standpoint. For this reason, the US Food and Drug Administration has recently removed rapidly improving or minor stroke symptoms as a contraindication for thrombolysis.

This patient was young and worked as an engineer. Hand weakness would have been disabling for him. For these reasons, this patient was treated with IV tPA at 1 hour 55 minutes. His MRI showed two small punctate infarcts with one in the hand region of the motor cortex (Figure 4.1).

It should also be noted which antithrombotic agents will be used for secondary stroke prevention in this patient with minor stroke. If no cardioembolic mechanism of stroke is identified, which would require anticoagulation, this patient may potentially benefit from a short-term course of dual antiplatelet agents. In the CHANCE trial, 5170 Chinese patients with recent minor stroke or high-risk transient ischemic attack were randomized to a 21-day course of aspirin 75 mg and clopidogrel 75 mg or to aspirin alone. Patients treated with dual agents had significantly fewer strokes on 90-day follow-up (8.2% vs. 11.7%), without an increase in major bleeding events or intracranial hemorrhage. A trial evaluating

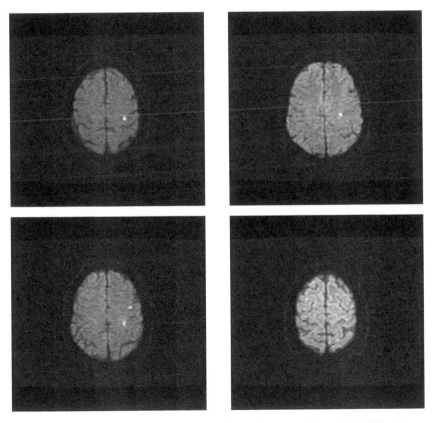

FIGURE 4.1 MRI diffusion-weighted sequence showing small punctate infarcts in the left frontal cortex.

dual antiplatelet therapy in the United States is currently underway to confirm the findings of CHANCE in a Western population. Care would have to be taken not to start antithrombotics within 24 hours of tPA administration.

KEY POINTS TO REMEMBER

· There is no NIHSS cutoff for IV tPA.
· Rapid improvement may portend early worsening, and more than one-fourth of patients with minor stroke are dependent on discharge if untreated.
· Rates of hemorrhage post-thrombolysis are low in minor stroke patients.
· It is reasonable to consider short-term dual antiplatelet therapy for patients with recent minor stroke or high-risk transient ischemic attack.

Further Reading

NINDS t-PA Stroke Study Group. Intracerebral hemorrhage after intravenous t-PA therapy for ischemic stroke. *Stroke* 1997;28(11):2109–2118.

Rajajee V, Kidwell C, Starkman S, et al. Early MRI and outcomes of untreated patients with mild or improving ischemic stroke. *Neurology* 2006;67:980.

Romano JG, Smith EE, Liang L, et al. Outcomes in mild acute ischemic stroke treated with intravenous thrombolysis: A retrospective analysis of the Get with the Guidelines–Stroke Registry. *JAMA Neurol* 2015;72(4):423–431.

Smith EE, Abdullah AR, Petkovska I, et al. Poor outcomes in patients who do not receive intravenous tissue plasminogen activator because of mild or improving ischemic stroke. *Stroke* 2005;36:2497–2499.

Smith EE, Fonarow GC, Reeves MJ, et al. Outcomes in mild or rapidly improving stroke not treated with intravenous recombinant tissue-type plasminogen activator: Findings from Get with the Guidelines–Stroke Registry. *Stroke* 2011;42:3110–3115.

Wang Y, Wang Y, Zhao X, et al. Clopidogrel with aspirin in acute minor stroke or transient ischemic attack. *N Engl J Med* 2013; 369: 11–9.

Yu AYX, Hill MD, Coutts SB. Should minor stroke patients be thrombolyzed? A focused review and future directions. *Int J Stroke* 2015;10:292–297.

5   Progressive Quadriplegia

A 68-year-old man with a past medical history of hyperlipidemia and prostatectomy for prostate cancer arrives in the emergency room via ambulance. The patient was walking to the bathroom in the morning and noticed sudden-onset diaphoresis, a band-like chest and back pain with associated right-sided weakness. In the emergency room, the patient progressed to have left arm and leg weakness as well, and he was found on examination to have numbness from the level of his clavicle downward. The patient was eventually intubated in the emergency room for hypoxia. A CT of the brain was unremarkable. The patient reports that his symptom onset was within the past 60 minutes.

What do you do now?

ACUTE MANAGEMENT AND WORKUP OF SPINAL CORD ISCHEMIA

A patient with acute-onset quadriparesis and sensory level raises suspicion for spinal cord ischemia. Unfortunately, given the rarity of the disease and the typical delay in making this difficult diagnosis in the acute setting, there are no standard protocols that dictate the acute management of nonsurgical spinal cord infarcts presenting to the emergency room. However, there are several issues that should be considered when deciding on emergency treatment, particularly intravenous thrombolysis (Box 5.1).

It is imperative to first consider the possibility of brainstem ischemia, which could also present with bilateral numbness and weakness. Such cases of brainstem stroke would be eligible for intravenous thrombolysis if presenting within a 4.5-hour window. After careful examination, if there remains uncertainty whether a patient is suffering brainstem or spinal cord injury due to a lack of localizing signs, CT angiogram (CTA) may help distinguish between the two. For instance, brainstem ischemia could be demonstrated if a basilar occlusion is identified. On the other hand, the same CTA could point to a potential source of spinal cord ischemia, such as aortic arch or vertebral artery dissection. Therefore, it is important to include imaging of the aortic arch and the descending aorta to rule out dissection, particularly in patients who present with accompanying back or chest pain, because this would be a contraindication to systemic thrombolysis. Our patient was found to have a sensory level on examination, indicative of spinal cord pathology, and an emergent CTA was performed to rule out aortic dissection. It is important to note that there are various mimics of spinal cord ischemia that may increase the risk of, or contraindicate, intravenous thrombolysis. This may necessitate emergent spinal imaging, particularly with MRI, to either (1) rule in ischemia by demonstrating restricted diffusion within the cord or (2) rule out compressive myelopathy due

---

BOX 5.1 **Suggested Emergency Diagnostic Evaluation of Acute Spinal Cord Infarct**

Noncontrast head CT
  Rule out intracranial hemorrhage
CTA head and neck
  Assess for vertebrobasilar occlusion
  Evaluate for aortic dissection
MRI Cspine
  Exclude epidural hematoma/neoplasm
  Detect infarction

---

to epidural hematomas, vascular malformations such as dural fistulas, or certain spinal tumors that could result in increased risk of bleeding. Spinal cord MRI has been reported to detect restricted diffusion on diffusion-weighted imaging (DWI) and apparent diffusion coefficient (ADC) maps in ischemia with high yield. Finally, if stroke is not confirmed on MRI, patients should be considered for other causes of acute myelopathy, such as neoplastic, infectious, and inflammatory diseases.

The spinal cord is supplied by one anterior and two posterior spinal arteries, which extend longitudinally along the surface of the cord in a variable manner. The anterior spinal artery arises from the intracranial vertebral artery and in the cervical region receives further supply from radicular arteries originating off the vertebral artery at the C3 level. The majority of spinal cord infarcts involve the anterior spinal artery, and the vascular anatomy described previously demonstrates how vertebral artery pathology could contribute to infarcts of the cervical spine. Ischemia more often affects the thoracic and lumbar spine based on arterial supply and resultant watershed regions; however, cervical cord infarcts can be seen 20% of the time. Our patient was eventually discovered on CTA to have degenerative spinal changes leading to facet joint hypertrophy resulting in compression, stenosis, and suspected dissection of the vertebral artery at the level of C5–C6. This was likely the causative etiology of his stroke (Box 5.2).

The clinical presentation of spinal cord infarction is typically acute, but it has often been described to progress over minutes to hours. Unilateral weakness can extend to quadriparesis, as was witnessed in this patient. Back pain at the level of the injury is common at presentation. The anterior spinal artery syndrome comprises the most common set of presenting symptoms of spinal cord infarct (seen in two-thirds of cases); it involves weakness and loss of temperature and pinprick sensation below the level of the lesion due to involvement of the corticospinal and spinothalamic tracts. However, vibration and proprioception sensation is typically spared unless the dorsal columns are affected by occlusion

---

BOX 5.2 **Causes of Spinal Cord Infarction**

Atherosclerosis of aorta or vertebral artery
Dissection of aorta or vertebral artery
Aortic surgery
Systemic hypotension
Vasculitis
Vascular malformations
No etiology identified in 28% of patients

of the posterior spinal artery. Other cord syndromes can be seen with spinal cord ischemia, such as Brown–Sequard syndrome, central cord syndrome, and cord transection. Approximately half of patients experience clinical improvement following cord infarction, with better rates of recovery in those presenting with less severe symptoms or those who begin to show early improvement. Of these patients, 40% recover the ability to walk independently, and 20% remain wheelchair-bound. Chronic bladder dysfunction is common, and acute respiratory compromise and hemodynamic instability are possible depending on the location of the stroke.

Few clinical data are available on the treatment of this disease outside of case reports and series. Reports of intravenous and intra-arterial thrombolysis have been published without showing significant adverse events. Other reports suggest varied treatment options such as corticosteroids or hyperbaric oxygen, but these have not been studied in a rigorous manner and are not recommended for routine clinical use. A large proportion of our experience with the disease is taken from cases following aortic surgeries, and institutional protocols have been published for spinal cord ischemia as a surgical complication. Perioperative interventions include the placement of lumbar drains and the use of pressor support to assist in increasing cord perfusion. Either of these interventions could potentially be dangerous in the setting of intravenous thrombolysis, and they have not been considered routine practice for nonsurgical patients presenting to the emergency department.

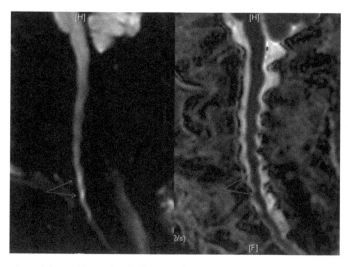

FIGURE 5.1 Acute infarct with restricted diffusion (left, DWI; right, ADC) within the anterior aspect of the spinal cord extending from C5 to T1.

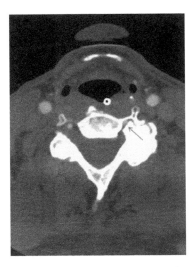

FIGURE 5.2 CT angiogram showing focal moderate stenosis of the left vertebral artery secondary to left-sided facet arthropathy with hypertrophy at the C5–C6 level.

Regardless of the acute management of these patients, they should still be treated with appropriate secondary stroke prevention. Therefore, all patients with spinal cord ischemia should undergo a routine stroke workup, in addition to being considered for specialized testing to evaluate for the cause of the spinal infarct, such as spinal angiography and serological and cerebrospinal fluid analysis to rule out infectious or inflammatory causes of vasculitis, and possibly hypercoagulable testing for patients who are young and for whom the cause of the infarct is otherwise unknown. Secondary prevention strategies are aimed at the mechanism of the stroke; for instance, antiplatelets are used in atherosclerotic mechanisms, and anticoagulation is employed if a high-risk cardioembolic etiology is identified. Statins should be started at similar dosing as that for cerebral ischemia. If a vascular malformation was identified during the evaluation, appropriate surgical management would be advised.

Our patient underwent emergent spinal MRI, which showed an extensive C5–T1 infarct in the anterior cord and no evidence of spinal hematoma (Figures 5.1 and 5.2). CTA ruled out aortic dissection, but it did note facet arthropathy at the C5–C6 level resulting in compression and stenosis of the vertebral artery. The patient was treated with full-dose IV tPA and was noted to make some modest improvement in terms of recovery of strength on the left side. However, 6 months later, the patient was still unable to walk independently.

- Spinal cord infarcts are rare, and no randomized trials are available to standardize their acute management.
- Most spinal cord infarcts involve the anterior spinal artery.
- Medical treatment for secondary stroke prevention should be focused on the stroke mechanism after a thorough stroke workup.
- Patients presenting with symptoms of spinal cord ischemia may be considered for pharmacological thrombolysis if they do not meet any of the standard exclusionary criteria, but experience with acute treatment of spinal cord ischemia is limited to case reports and series.
- Prior to administering tPA to a patient with spinal cord ischemia, the following tests should be obtained emergently: noncontrast head CT, noninvasive angiography to rule out aortic dissection, and spinal imaging (preferably MRI) to rule in ischemia or to rule out mimics that could make thrombolysis dangerous.

Further Reading

Cheung AT, Weiss SJ, McGarvey ML, et al. Interventions for reversing delayed-onset postoperative paraplegia after thoracic aortic reconstruction. *Ann Thorac Surg* 2002;74(2):413.

Lee K, Strozyk D, Rahman C, et al. Acute spinal cord ischemia: Treatment with intravenous and intra-arterial thrombolysis, hyperbaric, oxygen and hypothermia. *Cerebrovasc Dis* 2010;29:95–98.

Nedeltchev K, Loher TJ, Stepper F, et al. Long-term outcome of acute spinal cord ischemia syndrome. *Stroke* 2004;35(2):560.

Nogueira RG, Ferreira R, Grant PE, et al. Restricted diffusion in spinal cord infarction demonstrated by magnetic resonance line scan diffusion imaging. *Stroke* 2012;43(2):532–535.

Novy J, Caruzzo A, Maeder P, et al. Spinal cord ischemia: Clinical and imaging patterns, pathogenesis, and outcomes in 27 patients. *Arch Neurol* 2006;63(8):1113.

6 Malignant Edema

A 69-year-old man with hypertension and atrial fibrillation,
but not on anticoagulation, was evaluated for acute left
hemiparesis. The patient was found on the floor by the dog
walker. The time of onset was unknown. He was brought to
the emergency room and found to have left neglect, right
gaze deviation, left facial droop, and left hemiplegia. His
initial head CT showed a hyperdense right middle cerebral
artery (RMCA) sign and early infarct in the complete
RMCA territory. He developed increasing somnolence
over the following 2 days, and a CT scan 3 days after
admission showed increasing mass effect and midline
shift (Figure 6.1).

What do you do now?

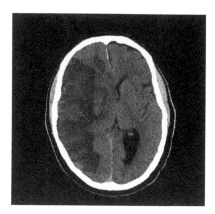

FIGURE 6.1 CT scan showing infarction of the complete RMCA territory with edema causing compression of the right lateral ventricle and shift of midline structures to the left.

SURGICAL DECOMPRESSION FOR LARGE MIDDLE CEREBRAL ARTERY AND CEREBELLAR STROKES

This is a patient with a malignant RMCA stroke. He has clinical signs of the full MCA territory being infarcted, and his imaging is consistent with this. It is important to recognize malignant MCA syndromes because there is high associated early worsening and death (up to 80%). Predictors of a malignant pattern include high initial NIHSS, usually greater than 16; younger age (less atrophy and room for swelling); and early signs of edema.

The cascade of deterioration is due to edema. Edema is usually maximal in 48–72 hours after a stroke. Because the skull is a rigid, confined space, there is little room to accommodate extra mass from brain edema. Shifting of normal brain occurs as in this patient. His CT shows compression of the right lateral ventricle and left shift with subfalcine herniation. However, the most morbid herniation pattern is transtentorial. The uncus of the temporal lobe can shift downward and compress the brainstem, leading to brainstem dysfunction and death.

Medical therapy includes intubation and intensive care unit (ICU) monitoring, preferably in a specialized ICU for neurological disease. Hyperosmolar therapy with mannitol or hypertonic saline is often used to reduce brain edema. The goal of these therapies is to reduce edema by drawing fluid intravascularly. Hypothermia is another modality being evaluated for reducing edema.

Another approach to relieve elevated intracranial pressure is hemicraniectomy. By removing the skull, edematous brain contents may herniate outward rather than compress other vital parts of the brain. There have been three European randomized trials of hemicraniectomy in malignant MCA strokes. All three were stopped early. A pooled analysis suggested benefit in patients treated within

48 hours of stroke onset and who were younger than age 60 years. This analysis found that 78% of patients treated medically died versus 29% with hemicraniectomy. A Cochrane meta-analysis also showed lower risk of death or disability defined as modified Rankin scale score greater than 4 with hemicraniectomy. However, the outcome of death or modified Rankin scale score greast3 was the same between the two arms. This suggests that patients may survive but with significant disability—unable to walk unassisted and requiring assistance for most needs.

A randomized trial also evaluated hemicraniectomy in patients older than age 60 years. In this trial, the median age of patients was 70 years, and similar effects were seen with greater likelihood of survival: 33% with medical therapy versus 70% in the hemicraniectomy group. Functional outcome results showed that the vast majority of surviving patients required assistance with most bodily needs. Unlike the surgical trials with younger patients, no patients older than age 60 years were independent 6 months after hemicraniectomy.

Similar to malignant MCA syndromes, rapid deterioration can occur with large cerebellar strokes. The posterior fossa has even less space to accommodate edema. Neurological worsening can occur due to edema with brainstem compression or compression of the fourth ventricle and resultant obstructive hydrocephalus. Progression to coma can be rapid.

Surgical decompression is a treatment option for large cerebellar strokes. Surgery is typically a suboccipital craniectomy to alleviate the increased intracranial pressure. In one case series of patients with cerebellar strokes and mass effect, there was a significant difference between patients treated with surgery and those who did not have surgery. Even 38% of patients in coma and posturing were nondisabled at discharge with surgery. Another nonrandomized study

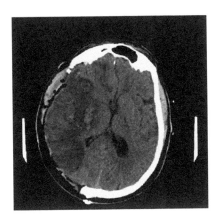

FIGURE 6.2 CT scan showing right hemicraniectomy with alleviation of mass effect on the left hemisphere.

of 84 patients showed that half of patients with worsening level of consciousness treated with surgery had meaningful recovery. However, there is a very short time window to intervene before neurological deficits may become permanent or herniation leads to death.

Hemicraniectomy was considered for the patient in the case presented in this chapter, who had a large, territorial MCA infarct. There was a discussion with the family, who stated his prior wishes for life-saving treatments. He was taken for emergent hemicraniectomy (Figure 6.2). He survived but required continuous care in a nursing home.

KEY POINTS TO REMEMBER

· Hemicraniectomy can be life-saving in malignant MCA syndromes.
· In cases of large, territorial stroke, careful discussions with family regarding the goal of surgical treatment should be reviewed because patients may survive with serious long-term disability.
· Quality of life after surgery requires further study.
· Patients with large cerebellar strokes need to be monitored closely for early clinical signs of elevated intracranial pressure.
· If there are signs of deterioration related to increased mass effect, surgical decompression needs to be considered with the goal of early treatment.

Further Reading

Cruz-Flores S, Berge E, Whittle IR. Surgical decompression for cerebral oedema in acute ischaemic stroke. *Cochrane Database Syst Rev* 2012;1:CD003435.

Hacke W, Schwab S, Horn M, et al. "Malignant" middle cerebral artery territory infarction: Clinical course and prognostic signs. *Arch Neurol* 1996;53:309–315.

Hornig CR, Rust DS, Busse O, et al. Space occupying cerebellar infarction: Clinical course and prognosis. *Stroke* 1994;25:372–374.

Jauss M, Krieger D, Hornig C, et al. Surgical and medical management of patients with massive cerebellar infarctions: Results of the German–Austrian Cerebellar Infarction Study. *J Neurol* 1999;246:257–264.

Juttler E, Unterberg A, Woitzik J, et al. Hemicraniectomy in older patients with extensive middle cerebral artery stroke. *N Engl J Med* 2014;370:1091–1100.

Searls DE, Pazdera L, Korbel E, et al. Symptoms and signs of posterior circulation ischemia in the New England Medical Center Posterior Circulation Registry. *Arch Neurol* 2012;69:346–351.

Vahedi K, Hofmeijer J, Juettler E, et al.; DECIMAL, DESTINY, and HAMLET investigators. Early decompressive surgery in malignant infarction of the middle cerebral artery: A pooled analysis of three randomised controlled trials. *Lancet Neurol* 2007;6:215–222.

7 To Treat or Not to Treat (Blood Pressure)

A 74-year-old man with hypertension, prior stroke, and coronary artery disease who had bypass surgery 20 years prior to presentation came to the ER with new left-sided weakness. He was found to have new left face, arm, and leg weakness. His blood pressure was 190/90. He was out of the window for IV tPA. His ECG showed an old right bundle branch block but no ischemic changes. The ER physician would like to treat his blood pressure.

What do you do now?

BLOOD PRESSURE MANAGEMENT IN ACUTE STROKE

Blood pressure and mortality after stroke follow a J-shaped curve, with both significantly low and high blood pressures associated with higher mortality. Blood pressure is commonly elevated after a stroke, and there is often an immediate impulse to treat the blood pressure. However, there are several theoretical reasons to *not* treat. Cerebral autoregulation allows for tight control of cerebral perfusion pressure over a wide range of mean arterial pressures. However, ischemic brain no longer has autoregulatory capacity, and the cerebral perfusion pressure is linearly dependent on mean arterial pressure. Therefore, abrupt lowering of blood pressure may reduce cerebral perfusion in ischemic tissue and expand the ischemic penumbra. Positron emission tomography (PET) studies support this. Lower blood pressures following stroke have also been associated with worsened stroke severity and comorbid coronary events.

However, sustained high blood pressure is also associated with increased mortality. Possible mechanisms may be an increase in cerebral edema or an increased risk of hemorrhage with elevated blood pressure. Also, in the IST trial, for every 10 mmHg increase in systolic blood pressure above 150, there was a 4.2% increase in recurrent stroke rates at 14 days.

A randomized trial, known as The angiotensin receptor blocker candesartan for treatment of acute stroke (SCAST), included more than 2000 subjects and did not find benefit in lowering blood pressure acutely following stroke. SCAST used candesartan versus placebo in ischemic or hemorrhagic stroke treated within 30 hours of stroke onset. The mean difference in blood pressure was 5/2 mmHg. There was no benefit for early treatment on the 6-month rate of stroke, myocardial infarction (MI), or vascular death; in fact, there was a trend toward worse functional outcome. In a more recent trial, 4071 Chinese ischemic stroke patients were randomized to permissive hypertension or early blood pressure reduction (initiated within 24 hours and achieving a target of <140/90 within 7 days). In this study, CATIS, the mean difference in systolic blood pressure between groups at 24 hours, was 9.1 mmHg and at 7 days was 9.3 mmHg. There was no difference in the outcome of death and major disability at 14 days or 3 months. However, in subgroup analysis, the authors demonstrated that patients who started blood pressure treatment more than 24 hours after symptom onset benefited with a significant reduction in death and disability at 14 days. These data largely implicate that there is no benefit of aggressive blood pressure control in the very early phases of stroke.

The American Heart Association recommends treatment for systolic blood pressure over 220 or diastolic blood pressure over 120. If treatment is warranted, the blood pressure should be lowered cautiously, 15% to 20% in the first 24 hours. A short-acting, easily titratable drug is preferred. Blood pressure often drops spontaneously within the first 24 hours without any intervention. Certainly, if there is evidence of end organ damage, such as acute MI, congestive heart failure, renal failure, hypertensive encephalopathy, or retinopathy, early treatment may need to be instituted. However, particular caution must be taken in those patients with arterial stenosis or occlusion and salvageable penumbra demonstrated on imaging.

This patient's blood pressure was not treated acutely and, 24 hours later, had spontaneously decreased to 160/80. He remained neurologically unchanged.

KEY POINTS TO REMEMBER

· Blood pressure is commonly elevated in the setting of stroke as a normal physiological response to cerebral ischemia.
· Acute lowering of blood pressure is not routinely recommended unless blood pressure is severely elevated (>220/120).

Further Reading

Adams HP Jr, del Zoppo G, Alberts MJ, et al. Guidelines for the early management of adults with ischemic stroke: A guideline from the American Heart Association/American Stroke Association Stroke Council. *Stroke* 2007;38:1655–1711.

He J, Zhang Y, Xu T, et al.; for the CATIS Investigators. Effects of immediate blood pressure reduction on death and major disability in patients with acute ischemic stroke: The CATIS randomized clinical trial. *JAMA* 2014;311(5):479–489.

Leonardi-Bee J, Bath PM, Phillips SJ; IST Collaborative Group. Blood pressure and clinical outcomes in the International Stroke Trial. *Stroke* 2002;33:1315–1320.

Potter JF, Robinson TG, Ford GA, et al. Controlling Hypertension and Hypotension Immediately Post-Stroke (CHHIPS): A randomized, placebo-controlled, double-blind trial. *Lancet Neurol* 2009;8:48–56.

Sandset EC, Bath PM, Boysen G, et al.; SCAST Study Group. The angiotensin-receptor blocker candesartan for treatment of acute stroke (SCAST): A randomised, placebo-controlled, double-blind trial. *Lancet* 2011 Feb 26;377(9767):741–750.

8 Unidentified Bright Objects

A 65-year-old woman with high cholesterol, treated thyroid cancer 4 years ago, and no history of migraine developed new-onset headache. She noticed right frontal episodic sharp pain. She had an MRI through her primary care physician and was referred for a stroke evaluation after MRI revealed an abnormality (Figure 8.1). Her blood pressure was 130/80, and she was neurologically normal. She would like to know how to prevent a stroke.

What do you do now?

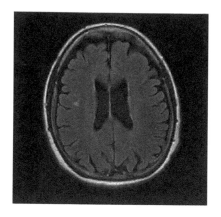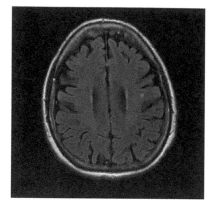

FIGURE 8.1   MRI fluid attenuation inversion recovery (FLAIR) with white matter hyperintensities.

PRIMARY PREVENTION OF STROKE

With the advent of more widespread imaging, subcortical white matter hyperintensities are increasingly being detected on MRI. One study of people aged 60–90 years found that 18% had silent infarcts on MRI. Follow-up imaging done on average 3 years later showed that 14% had new infarcts, most of which were also silent. However, other studies have demonstrated that silent brain infarcts can be harbingers of clinical strokes as well, with the risk possibly as high as five times that of patients without silent infarcts on MRI. Silent infarcts are associated with typical vascular risk factors: increasing age, high blood pressure, diabetes, high cholesterol, and smoking. White matter abnormalities have also been associated with cognitive decline and increased rates of mortality.

Although these white matter abnormalities were detected, this patient did not have a clinical stroke. However, because of the association between such imaging findings and vascular risk factors as well as stroke, an evaluation for vascular risk factors is warranted. She underwent imaging of her head and neck vessels as well as echocardiogram and cardiac monitoring. All results were normal.

In terms of primary prevention of stroke, patients should be screened for risk factors (Box 8.1). An international case–control study of 6000 patients discovered that 10 modifiable risk factors explain almost 90% of population-attributable risk of stroke.

Effective stroke prevention remains the best approach for reducing the burden of stroke, and methods of prevention should be directed at an individual's personal risk factors and overall stroke risk.

Hypertension is the most important modifiable risk factor for stroke. The risk of stroke is directly related to the degree of hypertension: The higher the blood pressure, the greater the risk of stroke. Multiple trials have shown the benefit of blood pressure control in all age groups and all degrees of hypertension. There are numerous agents to choose from, and angiotensin-converting enzyme (ACE) inhibitors, diuretics, angiotensin receptor blockers, beta-blockers, and calcium channel blockers have all been shown to lower the risk of stroke in various studies. There may be race/ethnic differences in response to ACE inhibitors, with one study showing higher stroke rates on lisinopril possibly due to less effective blood pressure control in African Americans. The choice of agent(s) can be tailored individually to the patient based on the degree of hypertension, sociodemographic factors, and the presence of other medical problems such as coronary disease or diabetes. The successful reduction of blood pressure is more important than the choice of antihypertensive.

All patients should have regular blood pressure monitoring and treatment for blood pressure higher than 140/90. However, there are data from randomized trials that show that patients at high risk for stroke may benefit from lower blood pressure targets as part of a primary prevention regimen. In the ACCORD trial, patients with diabetes at high cardiovascular risk were found to have significantly lower rates of stroke, a predefined secondary end point, if targeted to a systolic blood pressure goal less than 120. The SPRINT trial randomized hypertensive patients without diabetes to targeted systolic blood pressure control of less than 120 or less than 140. The patients with more aggressive blood pressure reduction experienced lower rates of the primary composite outcome of stroke, myocardial infarction, heart failure, or vascular death. Although there was no significant difference in stroke outcomes, there was lower overall mortality in the intensive-therapy group. Note that professional guidelines have not yet incorporated these more aggressive blood pressure targets into their recommendations. Furthermore, patients without previous stroke should be considered separately from those with a history of stroke, and it is possible that recommendations for blood pressure parameters in the future may differ between those being treated for primary versus secondary prevention.

All modifiable stroke risk factors should be evaluated for and addressed with the patient if they are present. Patients should be advised to quit smoking, monitored for serum lipids and glucose, and counseled on diet and exercise. Lipid management is particularly important to address with patients because statins have been found to be notably protective against stroke. In one large meta-analysis evaluating patients with elevated baseline low-density lipoprotein (LDL) cholesterol level, statins reduced the risk of all strokes by 21%. The most recent guidelines from the American Heart Association recommend calculating a patient's 10-year risk for atherosclerotic cardiovascular disease to guide treatment decisions on the intensity of statin dose. In patients aged 40–75 years, the following patient groups are all recommended for high-intensity dosing of statin: those with prior atherosclerotic cardiovascular disease; LDL cholesterol 190 mg/dL or greater; or at least a 7.5% 10-year risk of atherosclerotic cardiovascular disease, particularly if diabetes is present. It remains unclear if, and to what degree, electronic cigarettes are safer than traditional tobacco products in terms of personal and societal health risks. Specifically for women, hormone replacement should be avoided if a patient is at higher risk for stroke.

When risk factors are identified, patients often ask about their actual risk of stroke. Stroke risk assessment scales have been developed to estimate an individual's risk for stroke. These scales are based on collecting baseline data from a specific study population and monitoring over time for the development of stroke. Because these scales are based on the demographics of the population studied, the scale may not be valid for a particular person. For example, a scale based on White men may not be valid in predicting stroke for an African American woman. Despite such limitations, the Framingham Stroke Profile scale is widely used and includes a wide range of vascular risk factors. Points are assigned for various risk factors. This scale, among others, is available online for rapid calculation of risk. Alternatively, the American Heart Association and the American College of Cardiology have developed a cardiovascular risk calculator (available at http://my.americanheart.org/cvriskcalculator) that can be used to estimate the 10-year and lifetime risk of an atherosclerotic cardiovascular event.

The initiation of aspirin prophylaxis requires careful consideration of risks and benefits. Overall, aspirin (acetylsalicylic acid (ASA)) should be considered in patients who are at high risk of having a cardiac event. ASA for primary prevention of stroke in the general population is not well supported by epidemiological studies. In women, 81 mg daily or 100 mg every other day may lower the risk of ischemic stroke, especially in women older than age 65 years. In otherwise healthy people at low risk of a vascular event, ASA prophylaxis is not recommended. Any decision to start ASA as primary prevention should be weighed against the known risk of increased rates of both gastrointestinal bleeding and intracranial hemorrhage.

For this patient, using the Framingham Stroke Profile, based on her age and blood pressure, she has a 4% risk of stroke in 10 years. She was started on ASA 81 mg daily, and her blood pressure was monitored closely.

KEY POINTS TO REMEMBER

- Primary prevention involves careful monitoring and treatment of vascular risk factors.
- Particular attention should be paid to blood pressure, and antihypertensive therapy should be targeted to a goal of less than 140/90.
- Aspirin for primary prevention of stroke is not recommended in low-risk patients.
- Risk assessment calculators can help guide treatment decisions in individual cases, if the patient matches the demographics of the populations used to create the assessment tool.

Further Reading

ALLHAT Officers and Coordinators for the ALLHAT Collaborative Research Group. Major outcomes in high-risk hypertensive patients randomized to angiotensin-converting enzyme inhibitor or calcium channel blocker vs. diuretic: The Antihypertensive and Lipid-Lowering Treatment to Prevent Heart Attack Trial (ALLHAT). *JAMA* 2002;288:2981–2997.

Fanning JP, Wesley AJ, Wong AA, et al. Emerging spectra of silent brain infarction. *Stroke* 2014;45:3461–3471.

James PA, Oparil S, Carter BL, et al. 2014 Evidence-based guideline for the management of high blood pressure in adults: Report from the panel members appointed to the Eighth Joint National Committee (JNC 8). *JAMA* 2014;311(5):507–520.

Lawes CM, Bennett DA, Feigin VL, et al. Blood pressure and stroke: An overview of published reviews. *Stroke* 2004;35:776–785.

Meschia JF, Bushnell C, Boden-Albala B, et al. Guidelines for the primary prevention of stroke: A statement for healthcare professionals from the American Heart Association/American Stroke Association. *Stroke* 2014;45:3754–3832.

O'Donnel MJ, Xavier D, Liu L, et al. Risk factors for ischaemic and intracerebral haemorrhagic stroke in 22 countries (the INTERSTROKE study): A case–control study. *Lancet* 2010;376:112–123.

Rossouw JE, Anderson GL, Prentice RL, et al.; Writing Group for the Women's Health Initiative Investigators. Risks and benefits of estrogen plus progestin in healthy postmenopausal women: Principal results from the Women's Health Initiative randomized controlled trial. *JAMA* 2002;288(3):321–333.

Seshasai SR, Wijesuriya S, Sivakumaran R, et al. Effect of aspirin on vascular and nonvascular outcomes: Meta-analysis of randomized controlled trials. Arch Intern Med. 2012;172:209–216.

SPRINT Research Group. A randomized trial of intensive versus standard blood-pressure control. *N Engl J Med* 2015;373:2103–2116.

Stone NJ, Robinson JG, Lichtenstein AH, et al. 2013 ACC/AHA guideline on the treatment of blood cholesterol to reduce atherosclerotic cardiovascular risk in adults: A report of the American College of Cardiology/American Heart Association task force on practice guidelines. *Circulation* 2014;129:S1–S45.

Vermeer SE, Den Heijer T, Koudstaal PJ, et al. Incidence and risk factors of silent brain infarcts in the population-based Rotterdam Scan Study. *Stroke* 2003;34:392–396.

9 Detected Bruit

A 63-year-old man with hypertension, diabetes, high cholesterol, tobacco abuse, and coronary artery disease was referred for evaluation after being found to have internal carotid artery stenosis. He denies ever having had a stroke or transient ischemic attack (TIA). He had coronary artery bypass surgery 5 years ago and had carotid Dopplers at that time. He thought they were normal. He had follow-up Dopplers recently because of a carotid bruit detected on examination. These Dopplers now show left internal carotid artery stenosis >80%. He would like to know if he needs surgery.

What do you do now?

ASYMPTOMATIC INTERNAL CAROTID ARTERY STENOSIS

In a patient with asymptomatic carotid stenosis, one of the questions is whether revascularization is warranted. This is followed by what type of revascularization should be considered. There are two large randomized trials of carotid endarterectomy (CEA) versus medical therapy for stroke prevention that support the use of CEA in patients with asymptomatic stenosis. In the Asymptomatic Carotid Atherosclerosis Study (ACAS), the angiographic criterion of >60% stenosis was used. It found the 5-year risk of ipsilateral stroke, perioperative stroke, or death to be 5.1% with surgery versus 11% with medical therapy. The other trial, the Asymptomatic Carotid Surgery Trial (ACST), included Doppler criteria of 70% stenosis for enrollment. It found the 5-year risk of perioperative stroke, MI, death, or nonperioperative stroke to be 6.4% versus 11.8%. A follow-up study at 10 years showed the stroke risk to be 10.8% in the CEA arm versus 16.9% in the medical arm.

Overall, there appears to be a benefit of CEA in patients with asymptomatic stenosis. However, patients need to be selected very carefully. Subgroup analysis suggests women may not benefit as much from CEA. Age also plays a role because the number of patients older than age 75 years in trials of surgery is too few to establish efficacy in older people. Life expectancy must be considered because there is an upfront risk of perioperative stroke and death before a benefit may be realized. Choice of operator is also important. Any perioperative complication rates greater than the 2.3% for stroke or death reported in the ACAS trial could eliminate the potential benefit of the operation.

The other treatment option is angioplasty and stenting of the carotid stenosis. The Carotid Revascularization Endarterectomy Versus Stenting Trial (CREST) was a randomized trial of symptomatic and asymptomatic patients with carotid stenosis comparing stenting to CEA. In the asymptomatic patients, stenosis was >60% by angiography or >70% by ultrasound. The primary outcome was periprocedural stroke, death, or MI and ipsilateral stroke up to 4 years follow-up. No significant difference in outcomes (7.2% carotid angioplasty and stenting (CAS) vs. 6.8% CEA) was found. Perioperatively, stroke was more likely with CAS (4.1% vs. 2.3%), and MI was more likely after CEA (2.3% vs. 1.1%). Patients younger than age 70 years did better with CAS, and those older than age 70 years did better with CEA. Because CREST was not sufficiently powered to discern whether the treatment modalities were equivalent according to symptomatic status, a follow-up study called ACT I was performed on patients

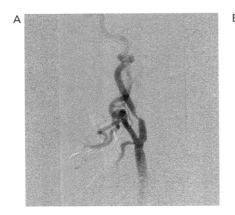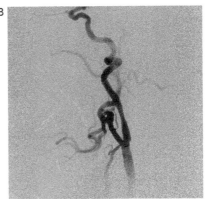

FIGURE 9.1 (A) Conventional angiography showing high-grade left ICA stenosis. (B) Carotid stent placed with improvement in stenosis.

with >70% asymptomatic carotid stenosis who were at standard risk for surgical complications and younger than age 80 years. There was no difference in the primary outcome of death, stroke, or MI within 30 days of the procedure or ipsilateral stroke within 1 year between the patients who underwent stenting (3.8%) and those who underwent endarterectomy (3.4%). The cumulative 5-year rate of stroke-free survival was 93.1% following stenting and 94.7% after CEA.

Overall, these studies suggest a modest benefit to revascularization in preventing stroke in patients with severe, asymptomatic carotid stenosis. However, medical therapy has improved over the years with better blood pressure control and wider use of statins. The benefit of CEA or stent versus current aggressive medical therapy is not known, and this is the focus of the currently enrolling CREST-2 trial. Patients should be selected very carefully for revascularization, and risks and benefits should be explained as discussed previously. Furthermore, patients who have progression of carotid stenosis, high-risk plaque elements such as ulceration, and microembolization detected on transcranial Doppler have plaque features that result in an increased risk of stroke and may thereby influence the risk:benefit ratio of surgical intervention.

This patient was young. He had been on good medical therapy after his coronary bypass surgery and yet had significant progression of carotid disease. He also had coronary disease and multiple medical problems placing him at higher risk for surgery. Given his age younger than 70 years and comorbidities, he had a stent placed without any perioperative complications (Figure 9.1).

· Select patients may benefit from revascularization of asymptomatic high-grade carotid stenosis.

· Carotid endarterectomy and endovascular stenting may be considered depending on the patient's comorbidities and operative risk profile.

· Stroke rates may be lower now from carotid stenosis because of aggressive medical management strategies.

Further Reading

Brott TG, Hobson RW, Howard G, et al. Stenting versus endarterectomy for treatment of carotid artery stenosis. *N Engl J Med* 2010;363:11–23.

Executive Committee for the Asymptomatic Carotid Atherosclerosis Study. Endarterectomy for asymptomatic carotid artery stenosis. *JAMA* 1995;273:1421–1428.

Halliday A, Harrison M, Hayter E, et al. 10 year stroke prevention after successful carotid endarterectomy for asymptomatic stenosis (ACST-1): A multicentre randomized trial. *Lancet* 2010;376:1074–1084.

MRC Asymptomatic Carotid Surgery Trial (ACST) Collaborative Group. Prevention of disabling and fatal strokes by successful carotid endarterectomy in patients without recent neurological symptoms: Randomized controlled trial. *Lancet* 2004;363:1491–1502.

Rosenfield K, Matsumura JS, Chaturvedi S, et al.; for the ACT I Investigators. Randomized trial of stent versus surgery for asymptomatic carotid stenosis. *N Engl J Med* 2016;374:1011–1020.

10 Small Vessel Disease

A 74-year-old man with hypertension arrives in the office 2 months after a hospitalization for dysarthria and ataxia. His hospital workup revealed a left pontine lacune. He was started on ASA and simvastatin in the hospital. On examination, his blood pressure was 150/80. He had a right facial droop, mild dysarthria, and slight right arm drift. His MRI showed a left paramedian pontine infarct. His magnetic resonance angiogram (MRA) was normal. His transthoracic echocardiogram was normal but had mild left ventricular hypertrophy. His low-density lipoprotein (LDL) and high-density lipoprotein (HDL) cholesterol levels were 140 and 39 respectively, and his liver function tests were normal. He is on an angiotensin receptor blocker (ARB) for blood pressure control. He would like to ensure that he is on the best medical regimen to prevent a recurrent stroke.

What do you do now?

SECONDARY STROKE PREVENTION AFTER LACUNAR STROKE

Lacunar strokes make up approximately 25% of all ischemic strokes. Lacunes are caused by infarction of a small penetrator vessel as a result of chronic arterial changes from hypertension and/or diabetes. Lacunar strokes are strongly associated with hypertension, particularly if this risk factor is poorly controlled. Because thrombosis occurs within small arteries, these strokes are subcortical; small in size; and typically located within the basal ganglia, internal capsule, thalamus, corona radiata, pons, or cerebellum (Figure 10.1). Based on the location of brain injury, a patient may have one of several classic lacunar syndromes, including pure motor, pure sensory, sensorimotor, ataxic hemiparesis, and clumsy hand dysarthria. Because lacunar infarcts often affect coalescing corticospinal tract fibers in the internal capsule, cerebral peduncle, or brainstem, motor weakness often involves the face, arm, and leg equally, contralateral to the side of infarct. However, the sensitivity and specificity of these clinical findings for lacunar infarct are not 100%, and a workup is certainly needed to exclude large vessel disease or a cardiac source of emboli. The imaging finding of a small, deep infarct in the absence of other possible stroke etiologies is strongly supportive of a lacunar etiology.

In this patient, a secondary stroke prevention strategy would need to include aggressive blood pressure monitoring and treatment. Several studies have shown that a reduction in blood pressure significantly lowers recurrent stroke risk. Although blood pressure targets need to be individualized based on patients'

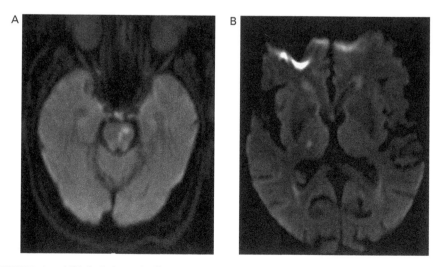

FIGURE 10.1 MRI displaying typical imaging characteristics of acute lacunar infarctions. Note small, subcortical infarcts in the left paramedian pons (A) and right thalamus (B).

comorbidities, current guideline recommendations advise a target pressure <140/ 90 in patients who have had a stroke. However, recent evidence from the SPS3 trial suggests that there may be some benefit from more strict blood pressure control (less than systolic 130 mmHg) in patients with lacunar stroke. SPS3 showed a strong trend toward reduction in the primary outcome of all stroke as well as significantly less intracerebral hemorrhage in those treated with more aggressive blood pressure control. The choice of antihypertensives also needs to be individualized. The use of ACE inhibitors or ARBs, either alone or in combination with diuretics, has been shown to be of benefit.

Statins are also important in secondary stroke prevention. The Stroke Prevention by Aggressive Reduction in Cholesterol Levels (SPARCL) trial randomized patients with stroke or TIA but no coronary disease to atorvastatin 80 mg versus placebo. Patients treated with atorvastatin had lower rates of recurrent stroke and cardiac events. There did appear to be a trend toward more hemorrhagic strokes.

Patients with lacunar strokes should also be started on an antiplatelet agent. Three medications may be used as first line: aspirin, aspirin with extended-release dipyridamole, and clopidogrel. There are minor differences in efficacy, so choice of drug is also tailored to the patient; the choice of agent may depend on cost, frequency of dosing, and tolerability of side effects. ASA is once a day and is usually well tolerated. For chronic secondary stroke prevention, doses of 50–1500 mg appear equivalent; however, there are greater gastrointestinal bleeding rates with higher doses. The typical dose prescribed is 81 mg or 325 mg. The combination of aspirin with extended-release dipyridamole when compared with ASA has a small benefit in secondary stroke prevention. However, headache and GI symptoms are more common with the combination, and headache more often leads to patient discontinuation. Clopidogrel and aspirin with extended release dipyridamole had similar efficacy for ischemic stroke prevention in the Prevention Regimen for Effectively Avoiding Second Strokes (PROFESS) trial; however, clopidogrel use resulted in less major bleeding, including intracranial hemorrhage. Alternatively, clopidogrel may have interactions with proton pump inhibitors, which may increase the risk of cardiovascular events. There are also genetic variants in hepatic metabolism that may make clopidogrel less effective in some patients.

Dual antiplatelet therapy with aspirin and clopidogrel has not been demonstrated to be beneficial in patients with lacunar stroke. The Management of Atherothrombosis with Clopidogrel in High Risk Patients (MATCH) trial, which enrolled more than half of its patients with lacunar stroke, showed that there were increased hemorrhagic complications in patients with stroke when placed on ASA and clopidogrel versus clopidogrel alone and there was no decrease in recurrent stroke rates. The regimen of ASA and clopidogrel was specifically tested in patients with lacunar strokes in the SPS3 trial. Patients with lacunes were randomized to ASA 325 daily versus ASA 325 and clopidogrel 75 mg daily. This trial showed no benefit of dual therapy: Recurrent stroke rate on ASA was 2.7% per year versus 2.5% per year on ASA and clopidogrel. However, there was a significantly increased risk of major hemorrhage and death on dual therapy. Given the potential for harm with long-term therapy, the combination of ASA and clopidogrel should not be used routinely in chronic stroke prevention if not indicated for other reasons (e.g., cardiac stenting).

This patient was continued on ASA. His statin was changed to atorvastatin. His blood pressure regimen was changed to increase his ARB, and follow-up blood pressure was 120/60.

KEY POINTS TO REMEMBER

- Preventing recurrent events after a lacunar stroke includes aggressive control of vascular risk factors, particularly blood pressure control.
- Antiplatelet monotherapy should be instituted with ASA, ASA with extended-release dipyridamole, or clopidogrel.
- Dual antiplatelet therapy with ASA and clopidogrel is associated with increased risk of bleeding and death.

Further Reading

Amarenco P, Bogousslavsky J, Callahan AIII, et al. High-dose atorvastatin after stroke or transient ischemic attack, *N Engl J Med* 2006;355:549–559.

Benavente OR, Coffey CS, Conwit R, et al. Blood-pressure targets in patients with recent lacunar stroke: The SPS3 trial. *Lancet* 2013;382:507–515.

Benavente OR, Hart RG, McClure LA, et al. Effects of clopidogrel added to aspirin in patients with recent lacunar stroke. *N Engl J Med* 2012;367:817–825.

Diener HC, Bogousslavsky J, Brass LM, et al. Aspirin and clopidogrel compared with clopidogrel alone after recent ischaemic stroke or transient ischaemic attack in high risk patients (MATCH): Randomized, double-blind, placebo-controlled trial, *Lancet* 2004;364:331–337.

Diener HC, Cunha L, Forbes C, et al. European Stroke Prevention Study: 2. Dipyridamole and acetylsalicylic acid in the secondary prevention of stroke. *J Neurol Sci* 1996;143:1–13.

Kernan WN, Ovbiagele B, Black HR, et al. Guidelines for the prevention of stroke in patients with stroke and transient ischemic attack: A guideline for healthcare professionals from the American Heart Association/American Stroke Association. *Stroke* 2014;45(7):2160–2236.

Progress Collaborative Group. Randomised trial of a perindopril-based blood-pressure-lowering regimen among 6,105 individuals with previous stroke or transient ischaemic attack. *Lancet* 2001;358:1033–1041.

Sacco RL, Diener HC, Yusuf S, et al. Aspirin and extended-release dipyridamole versus clopidogrel for recurrent stroke. *N Engl J Med* 2008;359:1238–1251.

Wright JT, Dunn JK, Cutler JA, et al. Outcomes in hypertensive black and nonblack patients treated with chlorthalidone, amlodipine, and lisinopril. *JAMA* 2005;293:1595–1608.

11 Obstructed Flow

A 68-year-old woman with a history of tobacco abuse
presented with left-sided weakness and dysarthria. She
had been having some difficulty walking at home but
did not seek medical attention. Her family noted a facial
droop and brought her to the ER. She was noted to have
a left homonymous hemianopia, left facial droop, mild
left arm and leg weakness, and some sensory neglect of
the left side. Her workup revealed a right middle cerebral
artery stroke and a high-grade right internal carotid artery
stenosis (Figure 11.1).

What do I do now?

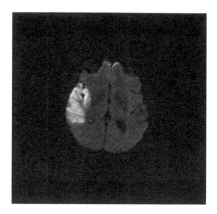

FIGURE 11.1 MRI DWI showing right temporal and insular infarct.

SECONDARY STROKE PREVENTION AFTER STROKE DUE TO CAROTID STENOSIS

Patients with stroke or TIA referable to a carotid artery with >50% stenosis should be considered for revascularization. The North American Symptomatic Carotid Endarterectomy Trial (NASCET) was an important randomized trial of CEA versus medical therapy in patients with symptomatic carotid stenosis. This study found a 2-year risk of ipsilateral stroke of 26% in the medical arm versus 9% in the surgical arm (including perioperative events) for patients with severe (>70%) stenosis. This is a dramatic absolute risk reduction, and CEA had been the standard of care for years. In patients with moderate (50–69%) stenosis in the NASCET trial, a more modest benefit of surgery was observed. The 5-year rate of ipsilateral stroke was 22% in the surgery arm and 16% in the medical arm. The risks and benefits of surgical intervention, and the individual patient characteristics, need to be heavily considered before referring a patient with 50–69% stenosis for CEA.

Angioplasty and stenting is now also an option for carotid revascularization, and there have been several randomized trials to support its use in symptomatic carotid stenosis. Most recently, CREST demonstrated no difference in the outcome of stroke, MI, or death between patients (symptomatic and asymptomatic) with moderate to severe stenosis who were treated with CEA versus stenting. Considering specifically the outcome of stroke, stroke occurred more frequently with stenting (4.1% vs. 2.3%). However, MI occurred more frequently with CEA (2.3% vs. 1.1%). Also, in the CREST trial there was an age difference, with older patients faring better with CEA and younger patients doing better with stenting (age 70 years was the cutoff).

There are many factors to consider in the decision for surgery. Operator experience is important. Surgical risk should be evaluated because advanced age, female gender, heart failure, active coronary artery disease, lung disease, and chronic renal insufficiency have all been associated with perioperative complications with CEA. Patients with unfavorable anatomy, neck irradiation, contralateral occlusion, and restenosis after prior CEA are also at higher risk of perioperative stroke and death. With stenting, perioperative stroke may be more common than MI. Stenting also requires dual antiplatelet therapy for the short term following the procedure.

The highest risk period for recurrent stroke is within the first 2 weeks. Thus, when possible, patients should be treated within this window.

This patient had low surgical risk and anatomy amenable to CEA. She had surgery 1 week after her stroke.

KEY POINTS TO REMEMBER

- Patients with symptomatic high-grade carotid stenosis with TIA or nondisabling stroke benefit from revascularization. The benefit of revascularization is more modest in patients with 50–69% stenosis, but it may be considered if patients are carefully selected.
- Either CEA or stenting may be considered depending on the patient's risk profile and anatomy.
- Treatment should be performed within 2 weeks, if possible.

Further Reading

Barnett HJ, Taylor DW, Eliasziw M, et al. Benefit of carotid endarterectomy in patients with symptomatic moderate or severe stenosis. North American Symptomatic Carotid Endarterectomy Trial Collaborators. *N Engl J Med* 1998;339:1415–1425.

Brott TG, Hobson RW, Howard G, et al. Stenting versus endarterectomy for treatment of carotid artery stenosis. *N Engl J Med* 2010;363:11–23.

Kernan WN, Ovbiagele B, Black HR, et al. Guidelines for the prevention of stroke in patients with stroke and transient ischemic attack: A guideline for healthcare professionals from the American Heart Association/American Stroke Association. *Stroke* 2014;45(7):2160–2236.

Mas JL, Chatellier G, Beyssen B, et al. Endarterectomy versus stenting in patients with symptomatic severe carotid stenosis. *N Engl J Med* 2006;355:1660–1671.

Rothwell PM, Eliasziw M, Gutnikov SA, et al. Endarterectomy for symptomatic carotid stenosis in relation to clinical subgroups and timing of surgery. *Lancet* 2004;363:915–924.

A 73-year-old man with hypertension and diabetes was
visiting his wife in the hospital when he developed acute
change in speech. He was noted to be speaking gibberish
and not making any sense. He had no vision, motor,
or sensory symptoms. The aphasia lasted 1 hour and
resolved spontaneously. In the ER, his blood pressure was
180/113. He was neurologically normal. He was admitted
for an evaluation for TIA and was found to have infarct
on MRI despite resolution of symptoms (Figure 12.1). His
cardiac evaluation for source of emboli was nonrevealing.
His CT angiogram showed intracranial atherosclerosis
involving the left middle cerebral artery (MCA) with
irregularity and narrowing but without focal stenosis.
He had evidence of atherosclerosis in the basilar artery
as well.

What do you do now?

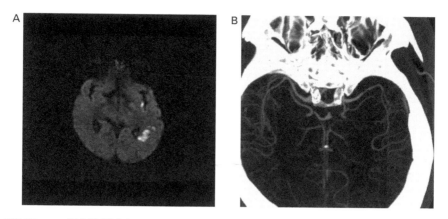

FIGURE 12.1 (A) MRI DWI showing patchy left MCA infarcts. (B) CT angiography showing irregularity and stenosis of the left MCA.

SECONDARY STROKE PREVENTION AFTER STROKE DUE TO INTRACRANIAL ATHEROSCLEROSIS

Intracranial atherosclerosis is associated with a high risk of recurrent stroke, especially with high-grade stenosis (70–99%). Recurrent stroke rates can be as high as 12–15% within 1 year, even with appropriate medical therapy. Asians and African Americans are more likely to develop intracranial atherosclerosis, unlike Caucasian patients, who typically develop atherosclerosis in the extracranial arteries. The arteries most likely to be affected by atherosclerosis, in order of descending prevalence, include the vertebral or basilar arteries, the MCA, the anterior cerebral artery, and the posterior cerebral artery.

The best preventative strategy in these patients has been debated in the past. Now, optimal medical management has been defined by randomized trials, and medical management has proven superior to surgical stenting of intracranial disease.

The Warfarin–Aspirin Symptomatic Intracranial Disease (WASID) trial was a randomized trial of warfarin (INR 2–3) versus aspirin (ASA) 1300 mg in patients with stroke or TIA and angiographically proven 50–99% stenosis of an intracranial vessel. This trial was stopped early because of a significant increase in death and major bleeding in the warfarin arm without additional benefit compared to ASA. Medical therapy for intracranial atherosclerosis now does not include anticoagulation.

Similar to trials of revascularization in the extracranial carotids, there have been studies of intracranial stenting to lower recurrent stroke rates in patients with high-grade intracranial stenosis. Registry data suggested there was a benefit to stenting with relatively low periprocedural complications. However, a randomized trial—Stenting vs. Aggressive Medical Management for Preventing Recurrent Stroke in Intracranial Stenosis (SAMMPRIS)—showed no benefit of intracranial stenting when compared to maximal medical management. In fact, there were significantly higher rates of stroke and death at 30 days in the stenting arm (14.7% vs. 5.8%). One-third of the early strokes after stenting were hemorrhages. Two important differences between the surgical treatment in the randomized trial and registries were that in SAMMPRIS only high-grade stenoses were included (>70%) and all patients had very recent (within 30 days) stroke. Therefore, patients in the randomized study may have been higher risk procedural candidates, perhaps explaining the difference in stroke and complication rates observed in the clinical trial and real-world practice. The results of SAMMPRIS were upheld in a recent, similarly designed trial using a different stenting device. The Vitesse Intracranial Stent Study for Ischemic Therapy (VISSIT) trial found that the rate of recurrent stroke or transient ischemic attack at 1 year was significantly higher following stenting than if patients were medically managed (34.5% vs. 9.4%), and the majority of these events occurred within the first 30 days.

In both SAMMPRISS and VISSIT, best medical therapy proved to be very effective. Observed rates of recurrent stroke in these trials were much less than expected from previous experience: 5.8% at 30 days and 12.2% at 1 year. In both studies, medical treatment was aggressive and included short-term, dual antiplatelet therapy using ASA 81–325 mg and clopidogrel 75 mg for 90 days. This particular antithrombotic regimen may have been important to the success of the medical management arm in these trials. Dual antiplatelet therapy has been found to reduce microemboli from symptomatic intracranial stenosis, and, in the Clopidogrel in High-Risk Patients with Acute Nondisabling Cerbrovascular Events (CHANCE) trial, short-term dual antiplatelet therapy lowered recurrent stroke rates in patients with high-risk minor stroke and TIA without increasing hemorrhage risk. Medical therapy in these trials also included aggressive blood pressure control that was targeted to <140/90 or 130/80 if diabetic, lipid management with statin for a goal LDL <70 mg/dL, diabetes treatment, smoking cessation, weight loss, and exercise. Based on the most recent American Heart Association guidelines, patients with stroke caused by intracranial atherosclerosis should be treated with high-intensity statin if tolerated. This includes atorvastatin 40–80 mg or rosuvastatin 20–40 mg. For now, such strict medical therapy is the most effective option for patients with intracranial atherosclerosis, and it is reasonable to consider short-term dual antiplatelet agents if the patient is not otherwise at excessive risk for bleeding.

· In most cases, intracranial atherosclerosis should be treated medically.

· It is reasonable to consider treating patients with short-term dual antiplatelets (ASA plus clopidogrel) following a stroke caused by an intracranial stenosis.

· Patients with stroke caused by intracranial atherosclerosis should be started on high-intensity statin therapy.

· Aggressive medical therapy is effective.

· There is a high risk of ischemic stroke, intracerebral hemorrhage, and death with intracranial stenting.

Further Reading

Chimowitz MI, Lynn MJ, Derdeyn CP, et al. Stenting versus aggressive medical therapy for intracranial arterial stenosis. *N Engl J Med* 2011;365:993–1003.

Chimowitz MI, Lynn MJ, Howlett-Smith H, et al. Comparison of warfarin and aspirin for symptomatic intracranial arterial stenosis. *N Engl J Med* 2005;352:1305–1316.

Stone NJ, Robinson JG, Lichtenstein AH, et al. 2013 ACC/AHA guideline on the treatment of blood cholesterol to reduce atherosclerotic cardiovascular risk in adults: A report of the American College of Cardiology/American Heart Association Task Force on Practice Guidelines. *Circulation* 2014;129:S1–S45.

Wong KS, Chen C, Fu J, et al. Clopidogrel plus aspirin versus aspirin alone for reducing embolisation in patients with acute symptomatic cerebral or carotid artery stenosis (CLAIR study): A randomised, open-label, blinded-endpoint trial. *Lancet Neurol* 2010;9:489–497.

Zaidat OO, Fitzsimmons BF, Woodward BK, et al. Effect of a balloon-expandable intracranial stent vs. medical therapy on risk of stroke in patients with symptomatic intracranial stenosis: The VISSIT randomized clinical trial. *JAMA* 2015;313(12):1240–1248.

13 A New Arrhythmia

A 55-year-old woman with hypertension and diabetes was hospitalized with congestive heart failure and was found to have rapid atrial fibrillation. Her heart rate was controlled, and she was started on warfarin. She was discharged home when her INR became therapeutic. The next day, she developed acute facial droop and dysarthria. She returned to the ER, and her INR on admission was 2.4. She was found to have some mild speech hesitancy and a right facial droop but was otherwise neurologically normal.

Her MRI showed a left frontal infarct with some small hemorrhagic transformation (Figure 13.1). She was discharged on warfarin. She returned for follow-up 2 weeks later and would like to discuss her options for stroke prevention.

What do you do now?

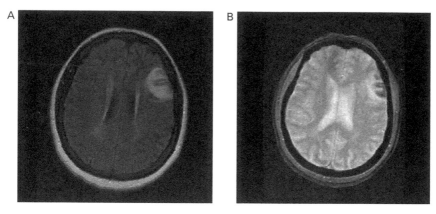

FIGURE 13.1 (A) MRI FLAIR showing small left frontal infarct. (B) Gradient echo sequence with hypointensity consistent with hemorrhagic transformation.

SECONDARY STROKE PREVENTION AFTER CARDIOEMBOLIC STROKE DUE TO ATRIAL FIBRILLATION

Atrial fibrillation is a potent risk factor for stroke. The $CHADS_2$ and CHA_2DS_2-VASc score are often used to risk stratify patients to determine treatment.

$CHADS_2$

C   CHF: 1 point
H   Hypertension: 1 point
A   Age >75 years: 1 point
D   Diabetes: 1 point
S2   Stroke, TIA, or prior embolism: 2 points

CHA_2DS_2-VASC

C   CHF: 1 point
H   Hypertension: 1 point
A_2 Age ≥75 years: 2 points
     Age 65–74 years: 1 point
D   Diabetes: 1 point
S_2 Stroke, TIA, or prior embolism: 2 points
     Female sex: 1 point
VASc History of vascular disease

A score of 2 or higher typically warrants anticoagulation on both scales because both are associated with increased risk of stroke (Table 13.1). Because patients

TABLE 13.1 **Annual Risk of Stroke Based on CHA$_2$DS$_2$-VASc Score**

Score	Adjusted Stroke Rate (%)
0	0
1	1.3
2	2.2
3	3.2
4	4.0
5	6.7
6	9.8
7	9.6
8	6.7
9	15.2

who have had stroke automatically receive 2 points, they are in a moderate to high risk category and should be treated. The CHA$_2$DS$_2$-VASc score has recently been favored for use in clinical practice because it incorporates more non-major vascular risk factors and thereby better discriminates stroke risk in patients with lower scores on the scale.

Several studies in the past have shown the benefit of chronic anticoagulation with warfarin for secondary stroke prevention in patients with atrial fibrillation. For years, warfarin was the only option for anticoagulation. Clinicians encountered problems with compliance and difficulty with tight monitoring and control of the INR with the narrow goal INR range of 2 to 3. Recently, new options have been studied and approved by the US Food and Drug Administration (FDA) (Box 13.1).

All the new agents are as effective or more in preventing stroke compared with warfarin. They also appear safer from a hemorrhagic stroke standpoint. This patient had a small stroke with a small hemorrhagic transformation. Two weeks after the stroke, warfarin was stopped and she was placed on dabigatran.

BOX 13.1   **Oral Anticoagulants**

Warfarin

Vitamin K dependent
Multiple trials including European Atrial Fibrillation Trial
(EAFT): Recurrent stroke 12% placebo versus 4% with warfarin
Requires monitoring, dietary restrictions, may have poor compliance
Reversible, can monitor compliance, inexpensive

Dabigatran

Oral direct thrombin inhibitor
Randomized Evaluation of Long-term Anticoagulation Therapy
(RELY): Stroke or systemic embolism: 1.69% per year warfarin, 1.53%
low-dose dabigatran, 1.11% high dose; hemorrhagic stroke: 0.38% per
year warfarin, 0.12% per year low-dose, 0.10% per year high dose
Superior to warfarin at higher (150 mg bid) dosing
Higher rate of MI, no significant hepatotoxicity
FDA-approved 150 bid; 110 mg dose not available in the United
States; gastrointestinal (GI) bleeding risk especially in elderly; renal
clearance; for CrCl 15–30 mL/min, recommend dose is 75 mg bid,
although this dose is largely unstudied in randomized trials
Newly approved reversal agent available (idarucizumab)

Rivaroxaban

Oral factor Xa inhibitor
The Rivaroxaban Once Daily Oral Direct Factor Xa Inhibition Compared
with Vitamin K Antagonism for Prevention of Stroke and Embolism
Trial in Atrial Fibrillation (ROCKET AF): Stroke or systemic
emboli: 2.2% per year warfarin, 1.7% per year rivaroxaban; ICH: 0.7%
warfarin, 0.5% per year rivaroxaban
Study cohort with higher CHADS$_2$ score than in RELY
Once-a-day dosing
Higher GI bleeding risk than warfarin
Reversal agent (andexanet alfa) currently being studied

Apixaban

Oral Factor Xa inhibitor
Apixaban for Reduction in Stroke and Other Thromboembolic Events
in Atrial Fibrillation (ARISTOTLE): Ischemic stroke: 0.97% per year
apixiban, 1.05% per year warfarin; hemorrhagic stroke: 0.24% per year
apixiban, 0.47% warfarin
Apixaban Versus Acetylsalicylic Acid to Prevent Stroke in Atrial Fibrillation
Patients Who Have Failed or Are Unsuitable for Vitamin K Antagonist
Treatment (AVERROES): Patients deemed unsuitable for warfarin,
compared apixaban with ASA; stroke or systemic emboli: 1.6% per
year apixaban versus 3.7% on ASA, ICH 0.4% in both arms
Reversal agent (andexanet alfa) currently being studied

Edoxaban

Oral factor Xa inhibitor

Effective Anticoagulation with Factor Xa Next Generation in Atrial Fibrillation–Thrombolysis in Myocardial Infarction 48 (ENGAGE AF-TIMI 48): Stroke or systemic emboli: 1.18% per year high-dose edoxaban, 1.61% low-dose edoxaban, 1.50% warfarin; hemorrhagic stroke: 0.26% per year high-dose edoxaban, 0.16% low-dose edoxaban, 0.47% warfarin

GI bleeding risk higher with 60-mg dose and lower with 30 mg dose compared to warfarin

---

KEY POINTS TO REMEMBER

- Anticoagulation is the most effective strategy to prevent strokes in patients with atrial fibrillation and should be considered in patients with $CHADS_2$ or CHA_2DS_2-VASc scores of 2 or greater.
- Newer agents now provide more options for anticoagulation.
- Dabigatran, rivaroxaban, apixaban, and edoxaban appear to be at least as effective as warfarin and have fewer intracerebral hemorrhage complications.
- New reversal agents (idarucizumab and andexanet alfa) are under investigation for the direct thrombin and factor Xa inhibitors.

Further Reading

Camm AJ, Kirchhof P, Lip GY, et al. Guidelines for the management of atrial fibrillation: The Task Force for the Management of Atrial Fibrillation of the European Society of Cardiology (ESC). *Eur Heart J* 2010;31(19):2369–2429.

Connolly SJ, Eikelboom J, Joyner C, et al. Apixaban in patients with atrial fibrillation. *N Engl J Med* 2011;364:806–817.

Connolly SJ, Ezekowitz MD, Yusuf S, et al. Dabigatran versus warfarin in patients with atrial fibrillation. *N Engl J Med* 2009;361(12):1139–1151.

Giugliano RP, Ruff CT, Braunwald E, et al.; ENGAGE AF-TIMI 48 Investigators. Edoxaban versus warfarin in patients with atrial fibrillation. *N Engl J Med* 2013;369(22):2093–2104.

Granger CB, Alexander JH, McMurray JJ, et al. Apixaban versus warfarin in patients with atrial fibrillation. *N Engl J Med* 2011;365(11):981–992.

Patel MR, Mahaffey KW, Garg J, et al. Rivaroxaban versus warfarin in nonvalvular atrial fibrillation. *N Engl J Med* 2011;365(10):883–891.

Siegal DM, Curnutte JT, Connolly SJ, et al. Andexanet alfa for the reversal of factor Xa inhibitor activity. *N Engl J Med* 2015;373:2413–2424.

14 Arch Disease

A 65-year-old woman with hypertension, hyperlipidemia, and coronary artery disease with prior stenting arrives in the emergency room with acute-onset left arm weakness and numbness that started 2 days prior and has not resolved. Her MRI of the brain shows two small acute infarcts—one in the right precentral gyrus and one in the right thalamus (Figures 14.1 and 14.2). During hospitalization, the patient undergoes MRA of the head and neck, which was unremarkable, and no atrial fibrillation was uncovered on telemetry.

The patient has suffered strokes in two separate vascular territories: The motor cortex is supplied by the anterior circulation and the thalamus by the posterior cerebral artery. This raises suspicion for an embolic source and prompts an investigation with transesophageal echocardiography (TEE). TEE shows a complex plaque with mobile components in the aortic root at the sinotubular junction, protruding 8 mm into the aortic lumen. The patient is already on aspirin and statin for her coronary disease.

What do you do now?

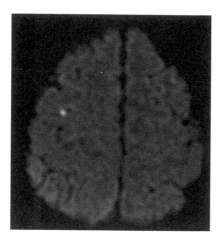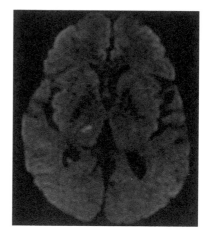

FIGURE 14.1   MRI of the brain showing separate acute infarcts in the primary motor cortex and thalamus of the right hemisphere.

SECONDARY STROKE PREVENTION AFTER CARDIOEMBOLIC STROKE DUE TO AORTIC ARCH ATHEROMA

Aortic arch atheroma is a manifestation of systemic atherosclerosis and commonly leads to thromboembolism in up to 21% of patients. The majority of these thromboembolic events include stroke and TIA, which tend to involve small and medium-sized intracranial arteries. Approximately 60% of patients older than age 60 years have some degree of atherosclerosis of the aortic arch, so

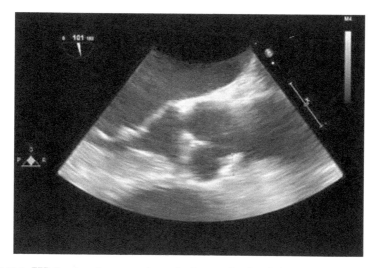

FIGURE 14.2   TEE showing a large, complex aortic plaque at the sinotubular junction.

it is important to identify plaque features that pose the highest risk for causing stroke and therefore warrant specific attention.

Aortic arch plaques are best identified with TEE, which has 90% sensitivity and specificity for detecting aortic plaque. A plaque is considered high risk if it is complex on TEE, defined as having one or more of the following elements: more than 4 mm in thickness, ulceration, mobile components, or high degree of protrusion into the aortic lumen. The strongest association appears to be with the size of the plaque: Recurrent stroke rates at 2 years are less than 4% if the plaque is <4 mm thick and up to 12% if the plaque is >4 mm.

It is important to rule out an alternative source of cardioembolism, such as atrial fibrillation, in patients with aortic atherosclerosis because this may necessitate secondary prevention with anticoagulation. However, in the absence of atrial fibrillation, warfarin has not been proven to be superior to antiplatelet therapy. The only randomized trial to directly compare antiplatelet therapy to warfarin in this setting was the Aortic Arch Related Cerebral Hazard Trial (ARCH). The ARCH trial compared warfarin (INR target range 2–3) to the combination of low-dose aspirin and clopidogrel 75 mg in patients with recent thromboembolism from complex aortic arch plaque. The authors reported a 24% nonsignificant relative risk reduction with antiplatelet therapy, and the following outcomes were noted only in the anticoagulation arm: MI, peripheral embolism, vascular death, and the need for salvage revascularization procedure. However, the study was halted due to low recruitment rates and was underpowered to make any definite clinical claims. Stroke rates in this trial were also much lower than expected (2.17% per year in the antiplatelet arm), which may have been a function of aggressive blood pressure control and statin usage in the study population. Statins have been shown to be independently protective against embolic events in complex aortic arch atherosclerosis. Similarly, hypertension and tobacco exposure are significant modifiable risk factors in this patient population, as they are in those with other evidence of systemic atherosclerosis. It is important to note that there was no antiplatelet monotherapy arm in the ARCH trial because this study was designed prior to the publication of MATCH in 2004. The MATCH trial demonstrated that dual antiplatelet therapy for long-term secondary stroke prevention is associated with a significantly increased risk of life-threatening and major bleeding compared to clopidogrel monotherapy. It is unclear if single- or dual-agent antiplatelets are preferable in patients with aortic arch atherosclerosis because this question has not been addressed in a randomized manner.

This patient was placed on dual antiplatelet agents with aspirin 81 mg and clopidogrel 75 mg because her embolic strokes occurred while on aspirin. She also was discharged on a high-intensity statin and had aggressive blood pressure control on follow-up. Despite these efforts, she was admitted 2 years later with recurrent stroke. Still, no atrial fibrillation was identified at this time. Although there are no randomized clinical trial data to support anticoagulation, her antithrombotic regimen was empirically switched to anticoagulation with warfarin because of the size and mobile elements of her persistent aortic arch plaque.

KEY POINTS TO REMEMBER

- Aortic arch plaques are considered high risk for embolism if they are >4 mm thick or have mobile, protuberant, or ulcerated components.
- It is unclear if antiplatelets or anticoagulation is superior for protection against recurrent embolism from aortic atherosclerosis; therefore, antiplatelet agents are typically started for initial stroke prevention given that they are easier to manage and have been used successfully in other models of atherosclerotic disease.
- Patients with stroke due to embolism from a high-risk aortic arch plaque should be treated with high-intensity statin, aggressive blood pressure control, and smoking cessation counseling, regardless of antithrombotic choice.

Further Reading

Amarenco P, Davis S, Jones EF, et al.; Aortic Arch Related Cerebral Hazard Trial Investigators. Clopidogrel plus aspirin versus warfarin in patients with stroke and aortic arch plaques. *Stroke* 2014;45(5):1248–1257.

Diener HC, Bogousslavsky J, Brass LM, et al; MATCH Investigators. Aspirin and clopidogrel compared with clopidogrel alone after recent ischemic stroke or transient ischemic attack in high-risk patients (MATCH): Randomized, double-blind, placebo-controlled trial. *Lancet* 2004;364:331–337.

The French Study of Aortic Plaques in Stroke Group. Atherosclerotic disease of the aortic arch as a risk factor for recurrent ischemic stroke. *N Engl J Med* 1996;334(19):1216.

Tunick PA, Nayar AC, Goodkin GM, et al.; NYU Atheroma Group. Effect of treatment on the incidence of stroke and other emboli in 519 patients with severe thoracic aortic plaque. *Am J Cardiol* 2002;90(12):1320.

Vaduganathan P, Ewton A, Nagueh SF, et al. Pathologic correlates of aortic plaques, thrombi and mobile "aortic debris" imaged in vivo with transesophageal echocardiography. *J Am Coll Cardiol* 1997;30(2):357.

15 Hole in My Heart

A 53-year-old woman with a history of hypothyroidism, hypertension, diabetes, and high cholesterol developed acute visual symptoms. She noticed loss of vision on the left side. She was initially seen by an ophthalmologist, who found a left homonymous hemianopia. She had an MRI, which confirmed a left posterior cerebral artery territory stroke. Her large arteries were normal. A TEE revealed a patent foramen ovale (PFO).

What do you do now?

SECONDARY STROKE PREVENTION AFTER CRYPTOGENIC
STROKE WITH PATENT FORAMEN OVALE

This is a patient who had a stroke, and an extensive evaluation did not reveal a large artery or obvious cardiac source of emboli. The infarct was not a lacune, given the involvement of the occipital cortex. An embolic-appearing stroke without an obvious source would be classified as cryptogenic. Approximately 30% of strokes are categorized as cryptogenic, but in patients younger than age 55 years, more (>40%) may be cryptogenic. Several studies have suggested an association between PFO, with or without atrial septal aneurysm, and cryptogenic stroke.

A PFO is a persistent communication between the two atria of the heart. This communication typically closes after birth, but in approximately 20% of people it remains open as a PFO. One possible mechanism for stroke from PFO is a paradoxical embolus in which a venous clot can traverse the PFO and enter the arterial circulation to the brain. Although studies have found an association between PFO and stroke, it does not appear to confer additional risk of recurrent stroke compared with cryptogenic stroke without PFO if on medical therapy.

The ideal medical therapy to prevent embolism from a PFO is not entirely clear. A subset of a larger randomized trial of warfarin versus ASA in stroke evaluated patients with cryptogenic stroke and PFO. In the PFO in Cryptogenic Stroke Study (PICSS) substudy, there was no difference in recurrent stroke rates between patients on ASA or warfarin. However, this patient population was older and had more vascular risk factors compared to other studies of patients with cryptogenic stroke. The PFO may not have been a significant contributor to stroke risk, so the results of this study may not apply to young patients with PFO and no other vascular risk factors. In a meta-analysis that included observational studies as well as the PICSS cohort, recurrent stroke rates were 1.3 per 100 person-years in patients on anticoagulation versus 3.2 per 100 person-years in patients on antiplatelet treatment, suggesting benefit of anticoagulation. There is insufficient evidence at this time to establish superiority of one medical therapy versus the other. This obviously does not apply to patients with concurrently documented indications for anticoagulation, such as deep venous thrombosis or hypercoagulable states.

PFO closure has also been considered in patients with cryptogenic stroke. The Evaluation of the STARFlex Septal Closure System in Patients with a Stroke and/or Transient Ischemic Attack due to Presumed Paradoxical Embolism through a Patent Foramen Ovale (CLOSURE I) trial used a percutaneous occlusive device to close PFOs. In this study, the 2-year stroke rate was 2.9% in the closure arm compared with 3.1% in the medical arm; there was no statistically significant difference. The medical arm received ASA, warfarin, or both at the investigator's discretion. The patients treated with PFO closure had a higher incidence of periprocedural atrial fibrillation. Two additional trials have since been published and also have not shown significant benefit of closure over medical therapy. In the Randomized Evaluation of Recurrent Stroke Comparing PFO Closure to Established Current Standard of Care Treatment (RESPECT) trial, although the primary intention-to-treat analysis showed neutral results, a prespecified analysis of patients who had completed the study per protocol demonstrated a benefit of closure (0.46 recurrent strokes per 100 person-years with closure versus 1.3 in medically treated patients). This is important because there were high amounts of crossover and dropout in these trials, which could complicate the intention-to-treat analysis. Benefit was greater in patients with larger shunts and atrial septal aneurysms in the RESPECT trial. Given the available data, PFO closure is not routinely recommended for secondary stroke prevention. Further data from ongoing trials may help determine if certain subgroups of patients can derive benefit from closure. Nevertheless, recurrent stroke rates in PFO patients seem to be generally low in the published data.

Other studies using longer duration cardiac monitoring suggest that there is a higher rate of paroxysmal atrial fibrillation in patients with cryptogenic stroke. It is important to remember to investigate other potential causes of emboli thoroughly, even if a PFO is detected.

This patient was continued on medical therapy with ASA, statin, blood pressure, and glycemic control. She had ambulatory cardiac monitoring for 2 weeks that did not reveal paroxysmal atrial fibrillation.

KEY POINTS TO REMEMBER

- PFO is associated with cryptogenic stroke.
- Medical therapy is favored for secondary stroke prevention, which may include ASA or warfarin.
- Currently, there is no evidence from randomized trials that cryptogenic stroke patients should routinely undergo closure of their PFOs.
- Patients with cryptogenic stroke should be investigated thoroughly for other possible stroke etiologies besides PFO.

Further Reading

Bogousslavsky J, Garazi S, Jeanrenaud X, et al. Stroke recurrence in patients with patent foramen ovale: The Lausanne Study. *Neurology* 1996;46:1301–1305.

Carroll JD, Saver JL, Thaler DE, et al. Closure of patent foramen ovale versus medical therapy after cryptogenic stroke. *N Engl J Med* 2013;368:1092–1100.

Furlan AJ, Meisman M, Massaro J, et al. Closure or medical therapy for cryptogenic stroke with patent foramen ovale. *N Engl J Med* 2012;366:991–999.

Homma S, Sacco RL, Di Tullio MR, et al. Effect of medical treatment in stroke patients with patent foramen ovale: Patent foramen ovale in Cryptogenic Stroke Study. *Circulation* 2002;105:2625–2631.

Kitsios GD, Dahabre IJ, Dabrh AM, et al. Patent foramen ovale closure and medical treatments for secondary stroke prevention. *Stroke* 2012;43:422–431.

Mas JL, Zuber M. Recurrent cerebrovascular events in patients with patent foramen ovale, atrial septal aneurysm, or both and cryptogenic stroke or transient ischemic attack. *Am Heart J* 1995;130:1083–1088.

Meier B, Kalesan B, Mattle HP, et al. Percutaneous closure of patent foramen ovale in cryptogenic embolism. *N Engl J Med* 2013;368:1083–1091.

Messe SR, Silverman IE, Kizer JR, et al. Practice parameter: Recurrent stroke with patent foramen ovale and atrial septal aneurysm: Report of the Quality Standards Subcommittee of the American Academy of Neurology. *Neurology* 2004;62:1042–1050.

16 Investigating the Occult

A 69-year-old woman with hypertension and high cholesterol is hospitalized with right-sided weakness and speech difficulty. She is found to have a stroke in the left MCA territory (Figure 16.1). She is in the hospital for 5 days, and no arrhythmia is detected on telemetry. Her large arteries are normal on MRA, and her TTE shows no abnormality. She is discharged home on aspirin and now follows up in the office.

What do you do now?

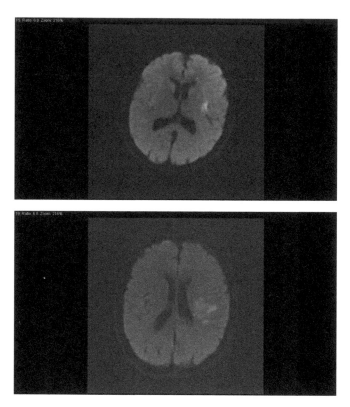

FIGURE 16.1 Embolic-appearing left MCA territory acute infarction on MRI.

CRYPTOGENIC STROKE WITH OCCULT ATRIAL FIBRILLATION

We evaluate patients for cause of stroke because it has implications for long-term treatment. Patients with stroke are subtyped into lacunar, large vessel disease, cardioembolic, other known cause (e.g., dissection), and cryptogenic mechanisms.

Cryptogenic stroke refers to those events of undetermined etiology despite a thorough evaluation. Unfortunately, cryptogenic disease comprises approximately 30% of all strokes. Cryptogenic strokes are nonlacunar, not due to large vessel disease, and no major cardiac source of emboli is found during a diagnostic workup. In these patients, recent studies suggest occult atrial fibrillation is more common than previously thought. Other suspected causes of cryptogenic stroke include undocumented hypercoagulable states, undiagnosed malignancies, and paradoxical embolization from a patent foramen ovale. However, given the size and distribution of this patient's stroke, an unidentified source of embolization is likely. Further diagnostic testing that can be ordered includes more intensive arrhythmia monitoring and a TEE to evaluate for left atrial appendage thrombus or aortic arch atheroma.

In one trial of patients with cryptogenic stroke aged 40 years or older, patients with an implanted cardiac monitor had atrial fibrillation detected at higher rates than those with a 24-hour external monitor within 6 months of stroke (8.9% vs. 1.4% in controls). More than 12% were found to have atrial fibrillation at 1 year. However, given the paroxysmal nature of the disease, it took a median of 84 days prior to the documentation of atrial fibrillation, and the majority of these patients were asymptomatic with a low burden of the arrhythmia. Nevertheless, the detection of atrial fibrillation in an embolic stroke patient is integral to secondary prevention strategies. For instance, in the CRYSTAL AF trial, discovery of the arrhythmia resulted in a change in management—the initiation of oral anticoagulation—in 97% of patients.

Another trial used an external 30-day event recorder compared with a standard 24-hour Holter monitor. This patient population was aged 55 years or older with cryptogenic stroke or TIA. The authors found that 16% of patients with the event monitor had atrial fibrillation at 90 days compared with 3.2% of the control group. Again, documentation of atrial fibrillation resulted in significantly more patients in the intensive monitoring arm being prescribed oral anticoagulation. The higher rates of arrhythmia detection in the 30-Day Cardiac Event Monitor Belt for Recording Atrial Fibrillation after a Cerebral Ischemic Event (EMBRACE) trial may be related to the older age of the cohort studied.

These studies confirm that in patients with embolic-appearing strokes, the likelihood of detecting atrial fibrillation is higher with more intensive monitoring. Suspicion for atrial fibrillation should be higher in older patients because this age group is more often afflicted with the arrhythmia. Detecting atrial fibrillation is important because it has implications for treatment: Patients with atrial fibrillation and stroke have moderate to high rates of stroke recurrence and therefore typically benefit from oral anticoagulation for secondary prevention if they are not at an abnormally high bleeding risk.

Because atrial fibrillation may be infrequent, short in duration, and asymptomatic, stroke patients should undergo aggressive arrhythmia monitoring if a cardioembolic etiology of stroke is suspected. Due to the erratic predictability of detecting atrial fibrillation, current research is pursuing more reliable biomarkers of stroke risk that may be easier to detect than occult arrhythmias. Also, multiple currently enrolling studies attempt to bypass the need for cardiac monitoring by empirically anticoagulating cryptogenic stroke patients who have a high likelihood of harboring occult cardioembolic stroke mechanisms.

This patient had a 30-day event monitor placed as an outpatient and was found to have paroxysmal atrial fibrillation without any clinical symptoms. Her episodes of atrial fibrillation events lasted several minutes. Given her prior stroke, she warranted anticoagulation for secondary stroke prevention. She was placed on an oral anticoagulant and has remained stroke free.

KEY POINTS TO REMEMBER

· Episodes of atrial fibrillation are often infrequent, short in duration, and asymptomatic.
· Patients with cryptogenic stroke should undergo intensive cardiac monitoring if suspected to have occult atrial fibrillation (particularly older patient populations).
· The longer cardiac monitoring continues, the more likely the clinician is to detect an occult arrhythmia that may be relevant to the etiology of stroke.
· Stroke patients with atrial fibrillation and embolic-appearing strokes on imaging should receive oral anticoagulation for secondary prevention unless they are at an abnormally high risk for bleeding.

Further Reading

Gladstone, DJ, Spring M, Dorian P, et al. Atrial fibrillation in patients with cryptogenic stroke. *N Engl J Med* 2014;370:2467–2477.
Sanna T, Diener HC, Passman RS, et al.; CRYSTAL AF Investigators. Cryptogenic stroke and underlying atrial fibrillation. *N Engl J Med* 2014;370:2478–2486.

17 A Horner's Syndrome Following Trauma

A 60-year-old healthy woman was brought to the ER with acute onset of global aphasia, left gaze deviation, and right hemiplegia. She had been seen in the ER 2 days prior to presentation after being struck by a car while walking on the street. She had a concussion, scalp laceration, and hand fracture but was discharged from the ER after normal CT of the head and cervical spine. At home, she had episodes of positional vertigo but was otherwise neurologically normal until the morning of presentation. She had witnessed onset of acute neurological change and was brought into the ER within 45 minutes of symptoms. She was found to have a left Horner's syndrome and signs of a large left MCA stroke.

Her head CT and CTA showed a dense left MCA sign and absence of flow in the extra- and intracranial left ICA (Figure 17.1). She had no evidence of hemorrhage or early infarct signs on the CT.

What do I do now?

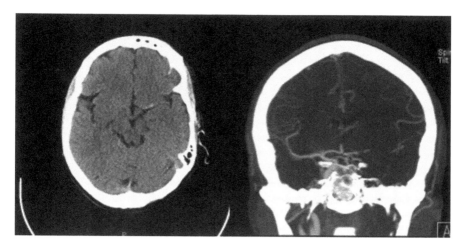

FIGURE 17.1 CT scan showing dense left MCA sign and CT angiogram showing occlusion of the left ICA.

CAROTID DISSECTION

Cervical arterial dissection is a rare cause of stroke, with an annual incidence of 2 or 3 per 100,000. Dissection of the cervical carotid artery must be considered in a patient with a history of trauma presenting with stroke and an ipsilateral Horner's sign. A dissection is typically due to an intimal tear allowing blood extravasation into a false lumen. This causes an intramural hematoma that can lead to vessel stenosis as well as compression of other structures. Alternatively, stroke can be caused by the embolization from a thrombus formed at the site of dissection. Ascending, third-order sympathetic fibers run along the carotid artery so that a dissection of the internal carotid artery is often associated with sympathetic dysfunction (Horner's syndrome): partial ptosis and miosis. Anhydrosis is typically not present with carotid dissection because the sudomotor fibers exit along the external carotid artery. Patients with dissection also commonly have headache or neck pain, sometimes as the only symptom of dissection. Hypoglossal dysfunction can also occur from compression of the 12th cranial nerve.

Dissections can be traumatic, as in this case, or spontaneous. Traumatic dissections may be due to relatively minor trauma or straining, such as with a fit of vomiting or coughing. Case reports have also described dissection after chiropractic manipulation and visits to the hair dresser with hyperextension of the neck. Spontaneous dissection has been associated with collagen vascular disease such as Ehler–Danlos type IV, Marfan's syndrome, and fibromuscular dysplasia. The etiology of most spontaneous dissections is not found. Given the often traumatic nature of dissection, it is a known cause of stroke in the young, with a peak prevalence in the fifth decade.

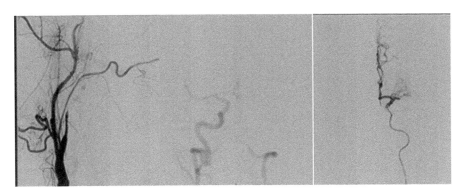

FIGURE 17.2 Angiogram showing tapering occlusion of the left ICA. Mechanical thrombectomy of the distal ICA allowed for cross-filling from the right.

Diagnosis is usually by noninvasive imaging. MRI with cross-sectional imaging of the vessel can detect the intramural hematoma. CTA can also show crescentic enhancement. On diagnostic cerebral angiography, one indication that a carotid occlusion is secondary to dissection is the flame sign, which is a progressive tapering of the visualized arterial lumen.

Although IV tPA is not contraindicated in patients with cervical dissection and stroke, recent head trauma is a contraindication. Therefore, this patient did not receive intravenous thrombolysis. Because acute endovascular therapy could allow for early recanalization, this patient was treated with mechanical embolectomy, which spared a large territorial infarct (Figures 17.2 and 17.3).

The prognosis is typically good following dissection, with relatively high rates of interval vessel healing and low rates of recurrent stroke. The majority of stenoses from dissection resolve within the first 3–6 months. In one case series of 161 patients with carotid dissection and severe stenosis or occlusion, 50 had persistent stenosis at 1 year versus 111 who recanalized. The annual recurrent stroke rates in these patients were very low, with 0.7% in the patients with permanent stenosis versus 0.3% in the patients with resolution of stenosis.

There are no data from adequately powered clinical trials to support antiplatelet therapy over anticoagulation or vice versa; as a result, no expert consensus has been reached on the preferred treatment of dissection. The best evidence we have for antithrombotic selection is from a randomized trial known as Cervical Artery Dissection in Stroke Study (CADISS). CADISS was a feasibility study not powered to be a definitive trial, so the results must be interpreted cautiously. A total of 250 patients with recent extracranial vertebral or carotid dissections were randomized to treatment with antiplatelets or anticoagulants. At 3 months, stroke rates were similar and very low in both arms (2% with antiplatelets vs. 1% with anticoagulants), and no patients died. The authors calculated that a

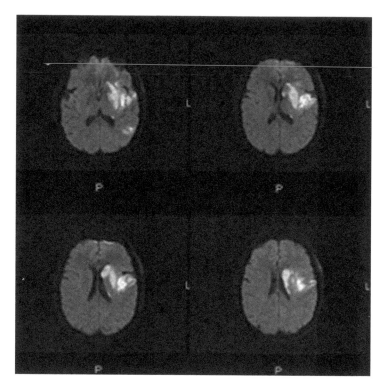

FIGURE 17.3   MRI with patchy left MCA infarct.

definitive study would require nearly 10,000 patients to complete; therefore, it is unclear if we will ever have an answer. However, given the confirmed low rate of clinical events following stroke, this may not be as clinically relevant a question as it once was. It is important to note that antiplatelets are cheaper, less difficult to manage, and less likely to cause bleeding side effects over long-term follow-up.

Real-world clinical practice varies, as evidenced by a survey in the United Kingdom showing that 50% of stroke physicians used anticoagulants, 30% used antiplatelets, and the remainder used both types of antithrombotics as the primary treatment for dissection. Although antiplatelet agents are most often used for asymptomatic dissections, many stroke experts treat symptomatic dissection with temporary anticoagulation for 3 to 6 months post-stroke, or until the vessel heals on follow-up imaging. However, because there was no increased benefit of warfarin treatment in both the CADISS trial and large meta-analyses of nonrandomized studies, it is reasonable to use an antiplatelet agent as an alternative to warfarin. Because recanalization can occur in the first few months post-treatment, most experts would typically repeat noninvasive imaging on follow-up to reassess the stenosis.

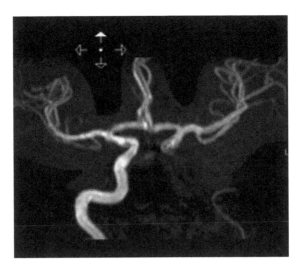

FIGURE 17.4 MRA showing persistent occlusion of the left ICA but robust collateral flow to the left MCA from the anterior communicating artery.

This patient was started on ASA and eventually treated with 3 months of warfarin. Three months later, she had only residual right facial palsy but was otherwise neurologically normal. Imaging showed that the left ICA remained persistently occluded, but she had robust collaterals (Figure 17.4). Her warfarin was stopped, and she was started on ASA. She has had no recurrent events.

KEY POINTS TO REMEMBER

· Stroke and a partial Horner's syndrome should prompt an investigation for dissection, particularly if accompanied by head or neck pain and recent trauma.
· Recurrent stroke rates after dissection are low on medical therapy.
· Antithrombotic therapy is typically used for stroke prevention. Either warfarin or aspirin may be used because neither has been found to be superior in recent studies.
· There is a wide variation in clinical practice, and some experts still recommend short-term anticoagulation for patients presenting with dissection and stroke. In routine use, antiplatelet therapy has been found to be cheaper, safer, and easier to manage than warfarin.
· It is reasonable to repeat noninvasive vascular imaging 3–6 months after initiating treatment for dissection in order to assess for vessel recanalization and healing of the damaged intimal layer.

Further Reading

Kennedy F, Lanfranconi S, Hicks C, et al. Antiplatelets vs. anticoagulation for dissection: CADISS nonrandomized arm and meta-analysis. *Neurology* 2012;79(7):686–689.

Kremer C, Mosso M, Georgiadis D, et al. Carotid dissection with permanent and transient occlusion or severe stenosis: Long term outcome. *Neurology* 2003;60:271–275.

Markus HS, Hayter E, Levi C, et al. Antiplatelet treatment compared with anticoagulation treatment for cervical artery dissection (CADISS): A randomised trial. *Lancet Neurol* 2015;14(4):361–367.

Menon RK, Markus HS, Norris JW. Results of a UK questionnaire of diagnosis and treatment in cervical artery dissection. *J Neurol Neurosurg Psychiatry* 2008;79(5):612.

Patel R, Adam R, Maldjian C, et al. Cervical carotid artery dissection: Current review of diagnosis and treatment. *Cardiol Rev* 2012;20:145–152.

Schievink WI. Spontaneous dissection of the carotid and vertebral arteries. *N Engl J Med* 2001;344:898–906.

18 Young Adult with Headache and Blurred Vision

A 36-year-old woman with a history of migraine presented with headache and blurred vision. She initially thought her visual symptoms were related to migraine, but symptoms worsened and she came to the ER. She was found to be neurologically normal in the ER. An MRI was done, and it showed small scattered temporal parietal infarcts (Figure 18.1). Her initial labs showed a thrombocytopenia and anemia. Her TEE was normal.

What do you do now?

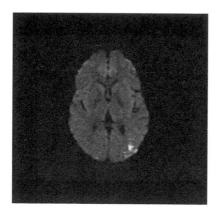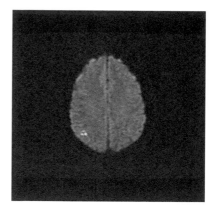

FIGURE 18.1 MRI DWI sequence showing recent bilateral infarcts in the temporal and parietal lobes.

STROKE IN A YOUNG ADULT

Stroke in young adults is rare. Typically, the definition of young in various studies has been under an age ranging from 45 to 55 years. Even in these young age groups, traditional vascular risk factors can develop and should be investigated. The prevalence of hypertension, diabetes, and high cholesterol has been increasing in young adults.

There are other risk factors that seem to be more prominent in young people. Dissection is a common cause of stroke in young. Cardiac sources of emboli are also detected in young adults, and these include prosthetic heart valves, endocarditis, cardiomyopathy, and cardiac tumors. Patent foramen ovale and atrial septal defects are also found more commonly in young patients with stroke. Other potential risk factors identified in young adults are smoking, migraine with aura, pregnancy and puerpurium, oral contraceptive use, and illicit drug use. An evaluation for stroke etiology should include screening for these mechanisms and is easily done by history. Vessel imaging and thorough cardiac evaluation are important as well.

There are numerous very rare causes of stroke, and these should be considered in the proper clinical context. Patients should be asked about systemic symptoms and other organ system involvement. A family history of venous or arterial thromboses is also important to obtain because this can indicate a hereditary thrombophilia. Evaluation for these more exotic causes of stroke requires more specialized testing (Box 18.1).

This patient was young and had no significant risk factors for stroke. Her initial workup included evaluation for more typical causes of stroke. Her TEE was normal. She had an angiogram that showed no evidence of large vessel

Specific Diagnostic Workup for Rare Etiologies of Stroke in the Young

Infectious

> Endocarditis: Erythrocyte sedimentation rate (ESR), complete blood count (CBC), TEE, blood cultures
> Tuberculosis: Cerebrospinal fluid (CSF) tuberculosis polymerase chain reaction (PCR), purified protein derivative, chest x-ray
> Syphilis: Rapid plasma reagin, CSF Venereal Disease Research Laboratory (VDRL), or fluorescent treponemal antibody absorption (FTA-ABS) testing
> Varicella zoster virus: CSF PCR
> HIV: Serologic testing
> Bacterial meningitis: CSF culture

Autoimmune

> Primary central nervous system angiitis: CSF cells and protein, cerebral angiogram, brain biopsy
> Systemic autoimmune diseases
> Systemic lupus erythematosus
> Sjögren's syndrome
> Behçet's disease
> Sarcoidosis
> Inflammatory bowel disease

Genetic

> Factor V Leiden
> Prothrombin gene mutation
> MTHFR mutation
> CADASIL: NOTCH 3
> Fabry's disease: alpha galactosidase activity

Hematologic

> Protein C/S
> Antithrombin III
> Hyperhomocysteinemia
> Sickle cell disease: hemoglobin electropheresis
> Disseminated intravascular coagulation (DIC)
> Thrombotic thrombocytopenic purpura (TTP)

vasculopathy. The key laboratory findings were the low platelets and anemia. A peripheral smear confirmed hemolytic anemia, and she was diagnosed with TTP, a rare cause of stroke. She was treated with plasma exchange.

· Stroke in young adults is rare.

· Although stroke may be due to traditional etiologies in this age group, other more unusual causes of stroke need to be investigated in the absence of traditional risk factors.

· There are multiple autoimmune, infectious, hematologic, and genetic disorders that can rarely cause stroke, and these etiologies are considered in a young patient with the appropriate clinical history.

Further Reading

Ferro JM, Massaro AR, Mas JL. Aetiological diagnosis of ischaemic stroke in young adults. *Lancet Neurol* 2010;9:1085–1096.

Larrue V, Berhoune N, Massabuau P, et al. Etiologic investigation of ischemic stroke in young adults. *Neurology* 2011;76:1983–1988.

19 Cancer and Coagulopathy

A 70-year-old woman with recently diagnosed lung cancer comes to the ER after being found by her husband with left-sided weakness. She was last seen by him 2 hours earlier in her usual state of health. On examination, she has weakness and neglect of the left side as well as a rightward gaze deviation. Her NIHSS score is 20. Her noncontrast head CT shows no acute findings and no intracranial metastases. The patient's husband tells you she was diagnosed with cancer 1 month ago, which was found to be a poorly differentiated adenocarcinoma of the lung with metastases to the thoracic spine. She is undergoing radiation to her spinal lesion, but she has not yet started chemotherapy. Although her vital signs are stable, she has a notable thrombocytopenia of 41,000.

What do you do now?

ISCHEMIC STROKE IN CANCER

This case illustrates that many patients with active cancer may have contraindications to intravenous thrombolysis based on either the direct or the indirect effects of their malignancy, or even the therapeutics aimed at treating their disease. This patient has thrombocytopenia below 100,000, which would preclude her from receiving IV tPA due to an increased risk of hemorrhagic complications. Her platelet abnormality is likely secondary to a coagulopathy imposed by her active cancer because she has not yet received chemotherapy. Little is known about the safety of intravenous thrombolysis in this patient population because cancer patients have often been excluded from randomized trials given their high rates of contraindications, such as bleeding diathesis, recent surgery, and brain metastases. Although this woman was found not to have brain metastases, a neoplastic brain lesion is a common reason why tPA is withheld in stroke patients. tPA has been found to be relatively safe in patients with benign brain tumors; however, there seem to be worse outcomes, including increased rates of symptomatic hemorrhage, in patients with malignant primary brain tumors. In a retrospective study of the Nationwide Inpatient Sample including 807 patients with cancer-associated stroke, patients with metastatic cancer did not have increased risk of intracranial hemorrhage following thrombolysis. However, careful consideration should be taken in any patient with brain metastasis, particularly those with primary melanoma or renal, thyroid, or germ cell carcinomas, which have the greatest tendency to bleed.

Patients with cancer have an increased risk of stroke; they comprise at least 10% of the stroke population (Box 19.1). Stroke may be the presenting sign of malignancy, with almost 75% of strokes occurring either at the time of or within 6 months of cancer diagnosis. Patients with adenocarcinoma, systemic metastases, or cryptogenic stroke subtypes seem to be particularly high-risk groups.

BOX 19.1 **The Most Common Cancers in Stroke Patients**

- Lung
- Primary brain tumors
- Hematological malignancies
- Prostate
- Gynecological
- Gastrointestinal (particularly pancreatic)
- Breast

Ischemic strokes may be caused by multiple mechanisms in cancer patients (Box 19.2).

Despite high rates of stroke in cancer, there is not much high-level evidence regarding the clinical treatment of these patients, with most of the data coming from observational studies and case series. In this population, treatment options should take into particular consideration the prognosis, goals of care, and the wishes of the patient and family. Intravenous thrombolysis could be considered in select patient populations presenting with acute stroke. In addition, successful outcomes have been reported following intra-arterial therapy in patients with active cancer and good premorbid functional status; however, these patients have not been studied in a randomized manner. Also, it is unclear what the optimum secondary prevention strategy is in these patients. A feasibility trial of enoxaparin versus aspirin therapy in patients with active cancer is currently in enrollment, but these results are not available. Therefore, it is suggested that the antithrombotic selection be aimed at the stroke mechanism. For instance, if a patient is found to have an atherosclerotic mechanism of stroke, antiplatelets should be considered first-line therapy. Conversely, if a patient has a cardioembolic mechanism of stroke, anticoagulation may be reasonable if the patient is not already at increased risk of bleeding, for instance, from cancer-related coagulopathy or hemorrhagic metastases. In patients with nonbacterial thrombotic endocarditis, also known as marantic endocarditis, there are some older data and expert opinion that these patients may benefit particularly from heparinoid products over warfarin. There is little experience with the novel oral anticoagulants in patients with stroke from cancer-related hypercoagulability because these medications are not currently approved for this purpose.

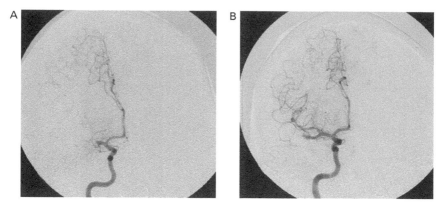

FIGURE 19.1 Cerebral angiogram displaying proximal right middle cerebral artery (M1) occlusion (A) and successful TICI IIb revascularization after thrombectomy with stent retriever (B); however, the inferior division of the middle cerebral artery remains occluded distally.

Our patient's thrombocytopenia was a contraindication to IV tPA. She was therefore taken for emergent mechanical thrombectomy after finding a proximal right middle cerebral artery occlusion (Figure 19.1). Following recanalization, the patient's neurological examination improved with resolution of her neglect and gaze preference but persistence of a mild left hemiparesis. Her repeat head CT showed only a small subcortical infarction and mild hemorrhagic conversion. Unfortunately, the next day the patient developed concurrent lower gastrointestinal bleeding and ST elevation myocardial infarction. Her blood work showed a D-dimer of 14,783 and fibrinogen of 134. Her laboratory studies and clinical thromboembolic events were consistent with a diffuse coagulopathy associated with her advanced lung adenocarcinoma. A bedside transthoracic echocardiogram demonstrated a small mitral valve vegetation indicative of marantic endocarditis. Marantic endocarditis results in strokes through multifocal cerebrovascular thrombosis and embolization from sterile platelet–fibrin cardiac vegetations. Of note, in patients with cancer and suspected cardioembolic stroke, transthoracic echocardiogram may be inadequate for identifying a possible or definite source of stroke, whereas TEE had a yield of up to 76% in one study.

The patient died 1 day later of cardiac arrest, after extensive discussions with the family resulted in the decision to pursue only palliative measures. The median survival following stroke in patients with active cancer at a large tertiary care cancer center was found to be only 84 days. Of these patients, 34% had recurrent thromboembolic events despite treatment, the majority of which occurred in the first month following the initial stroke.

- The coagulopathy associated with cancer is extremely high risk for ischemic stroke and ensuing mortality; the only definitive therapy may be treating the underlying neoplastic disease.
- Patients with active cancer should be considered for IV tPA in select cases; however, there are often contraindications. Intra-arterial therapy is reasonable to consider for these patients.
- Patients with active cancer and cryptogenic stroke should have D-dimer testing to assess for risk of coagulopathy and echocardiography to assess for vegetations from marantic endocarditis.
- It is unclear if antiplatelets or anticoagulation is superior in patients with active cancer; however, the secondary prevention strategy should be aimed at the presumed underlying mechanism.
- Prognosis, goals of care, and patient and family preferences should be discussed when considering treatment.

Further Reading

Cestari DM, Weine DM, Panageas KS, et al. Stroke in patients with cancer: Incidence and etiology. *Neurology* 2004;62:2025–2030.

Kim SJ, Park JH, Lee MJ, et al. Clues to occult cancer in patients with ischemic stroke. *PLoS One* 2012;7(9):e44959.

Merkler AE, Marcus JR, Gupta A, et al. Endovascular therapy for acute stroke in patients with cancer. *Neurohospitalist* 2014;4(3):133–135.

Murthy SB, Karanth S, Shah S, et al. Thrombolysis for acute ischemic stroke in patients with cancer: A population study. *Stroke* 2013;44:3573–3576.

Murthy SB, Moradiya Y, Shah S, et al. In-hospital outcomes of thrombolysis for acute ischemic stroke in patients with primary brain tumors. *J Clin Neurosci* 2015;22(3):474–478.

Navi BB, Singer S, Merkler AE, et al. Recurrent thromboembolic events after ischemic stroke in patients with cancer. *Neurology* 2014;83(1):26–33.

Navi BB, Singer S, Merkler AE, et al. Cryptogenic subtype predicts reduced survival among cancer patients with ischemic stroke. *Stroke* 2014;45(8):2292–2297.

Nguyen T, DeAngelis LM. Stroke in cancer patients. *Curr Neurol Neurosci Rep* 2006;6:187–192.

Rogers LR, Cho ES, Kempin S, et al. Cerebral infarction from non-bacterial thrombotic endocarditis. Clinical and pathological study including the effects of anticoagulation. *Am J Med* 1987;83:746–756.

20 Fevers in a Patient with Valve Replacement

A 74-year-old woman with hypertension, atrial fibrillation, and mechanical aortic and mitral valves presented with headache and confusion. A CT scan (Figure 20.1) showed intracerebral hemorrhage and a small amount of subarachnoid hemorrhage (SAH). Her INR is 2.3, and she is now neurologically normal. She was noted to have a fever with a temperature of 101.9.

What do you do now?

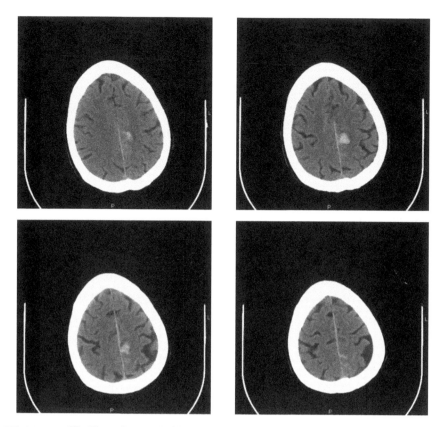

FIGURE 20.1 CT with small parasagittal intraparenchymal hemorrhage and small subarachnoid hemorrhage.

INFECTIVE ENDOCARDITIS AND ITS COMPLICATIONS

A patient with fever, mechanical valve, and a brain hemorrhage should raise strong suspicion for infective endocarditis. Neurological complications of bacterial endocarditis can be seen in 25% of patients. These complications include ischemic stroke, SAH, ICH, meningitis, abscess formation, and encephalopathy.

Stroke occurs from embolization of septic material from the infected heart valve and is very common in patients with infective endocarditis. Although the risk of stroke is as high as 9.1% in the month after the diagnosis of endocarditis, this risk is significantly elevated for months before and after the diagnosis. In endocarditis, intraparenchymal hemorrhage is more commonly due to hemorrhagic transformation of an ischemic infarct. However, rupture of a mycotic aneurysm may also cause ICH or SAH. Mycotic aneurysms are relatively rare

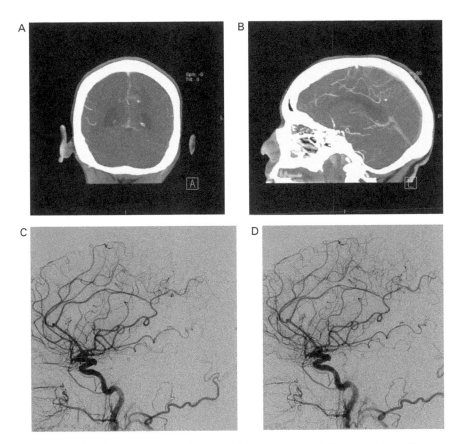

FIGURE 20.2 (A) CTA coronal view showing small left ACA aneurysm. (B) CTA sagittal view with distal left ACA aneurysm. (C) Cerebral angiogram lateral view of distal aneurysm. (D) Angiogram post-embolization of aneurysm.

and found in 2–10% of patients with infective endocarditis. Mycotic aneurysms arise from infective embolic debris that causes local inflammation of the vessel. Unlike berry aneurysms, mycotic aneurysms are not typically found at the circle of Willis because the emboli migrate distally in the arterial tree. For this reason, they are more difficult to detect on MRA or CTA.

Acute neurological deficit and abnormalities on imaging should be followed up with vessel imaging in patients with endocarditis. Noninvasive imaging such as MRA or CTA may be used initially. However, because of the small size and distal location, normal findings on MRA or CTA do not exclude mycotic aneurysms and conventional angiography may be needed. It is especially important to evaluate for an aneurysm in this patient, who will eventually need to be anticoagulated for her mechanical valves. We also evaluate for aneurysms in patients who need valve replacement because they are aggressively anticoagulated during surgery.

Best treatment for mycotic aneurysms is not clear. There are no randomized clinical trials. Based on several case series and expert opinion, ruptured aneurysms are usually treated with endovascular embolization or surgery. Unruptured aneurysms are treated medically with antibiotics and with careful serial monitoring for growth. If the lesion remains stable, antibiotics are continued, but if there is growth, treatment with embolization or surgery is considered.

This patient had a TEE, which showed no vegetations. Blood cultures grew *Streptococcus viridans*. She was started on antibiotics, and her warfarin was held. A CTA was done, which showed a distal ACA aneurysm (Figure 20.2).

Because this patient had a hemorrhage and she would eventually need to resume anticoagulation for her mechanical heart valves, she was taken for treatment with embolization. Her warfarin was held for 1 week and then resumed after embolization. She continued intravenous antibiotics for 6 weeks. A repeat angiogram at the end of her antibiotic course showed no new lesions.

KEY POINTS TO REMEMBER

- Fever and stroke or hemorrhage in a patient with mechanical valves should prompt an evaluation for bacterial endocarditis.
- Strokes are common in patients with infective endocarditis and may precede or follow a diagnosis of endocarditis by months.
- Mycotic aneurysms are rare but can cause hemorrhage. These aneurysms may require intervention with surgery or embolization if the patient is at risk for recurrent bleeding.

Further Reading

Heiro M, Nikoskelainen J, Engblom E, et al. Neurologic manifestations of infective endocarditis: A 17 year experience in a teaching hospital in Finland. *Arch Intern Med* 2000;160:2781–2787.

Merkler AE, Chu SY, Lerario MP, et al. Temporal relationship between infective endocarditis and stroke. *Neurology* 2015;85(6):512–516.

Peters PJ, Harrison T, Lennox JL. A dangerous dilemma: Management of infectious intracranial aneurysms complicating endocarditis. *Lancet Infect Dis* 2006;6:742–748.

21 Seeing Jellyfish

A 48-year-old man with a history of migraine since age
13 years presented with visual symptoms and left-sided
weakness. His migraines typically started with peripheral
vision loss and seeing "jellyfish" throughout the visual
field. This is usually followed by pulsatile headache. They
occur four times a year. The morning of admission, he
noticed his typical visual aura. However, this was followed
by left-sided weakness in addition to his usual headache.
He went to the ER. His visual symptoms resolved within
60 minutes. The weakness improved significantly, but
he was found to have a mild arm drift. He continued to
have headache. An MRI done acutely showed a region of
restricted diffusion in the right corona radiate (Figure 21.1).

What do you do now?

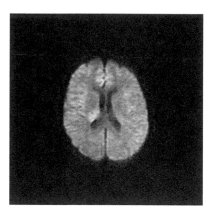

FIGURE 21.1   MRI DWI with evidence of infarct along the right lateral ventricle.

MIGRAINOUS STROKE

This patient is having a typical migraine attack with prolonged aura, but he has a new focal neurological deficit. As discussed in a prior chapter, migraine may be a stroke mimic, but migraine may also be a risk factor for stroke or, rarely, the cause of stroke. There is at least a twofold increased risk of ischemic stroke in patients with migraine. The association of migraine with stroke is especially strong in certain patient subgroups: women, the young, those who smoke cigarettes or use oral contraceptives, those with migraine auras, and those with a patent foramen ovale. Migraine has also been associated with increased burden of asymptomatic white matter infarct-like lesions, particularly in the posterior circulation. These are of unknown clinical significance.

There are many proposed neuropathological mechanisms linking migraine to stroke, and it is possible that these factors may cooperatively influence stroke risk in this population. During migraine, particularly the aura phase, there is alteration of ionic homeostasis due to cortical spreading depression as well as the release of multiple vasoactive chemicals such as endothelin, vasopressin, and serotonin. This can lead to vasospasm, oligemia, and a decrease in cerebral blood flow by 20–30%; alternatively, recurrent vasodilation may lead to impaired cerebral autoregulation. Release of similar vaso-inflammatory substances, both during a migraine and interictally, can result in endothelial change and increased platelet reactivity. These circulating vasoactive substances include endothelin, C-reactive protein, interleukins, and tumor necrosis factor-α.

Acute migraine can also directly cause stroke, although this clinical entity makes up fewer than 0.5% of acute stroke cases. The International Headache Society defines migrainous stroke as a typical attack of migraine, with aura symptoms persisting for longer than 60 minutes and with evidence of infarct on imaging in a relevant area of the brain. A study of patients with stroke in the setting of migraine included patients presenting with acute migraine (either with or without aura) and neurological symptoms, as well as acute infarct on brain MRI. The majority (70%) had DWI lesions in the posterior circulation consistent with acute infarction. Almost all (94%) had at least one other risk factor for stroke, especially hypertension. The exact mechanism of migraine directly causing stroke is unknown, but it is speculated that cerebral infarction is due to either sustained electrochemical changes during migraine aura or the release of vasoactive and inflammatory molecules that results in oligemia, vasospasm, and possibly thrombosis.

Migrainous stroke is a diagnosis of exclusion, and a thorough stroke workup is required to rule out more common, traditional stroke etiologies. This patient had a full evaluation of his vessels and heart, which demonstrated no evidence of a large artery or cardiac source of his stroke. He had no hematologic abnormalities. Because this patient had evidence of evolving infarct on imaging with symptoms occurring in the setting of a migraine, he was diagnosed with migrainous stroke. Although there are no clinical trial data to support this, migraine prophylaxis was initiated to reduce the frequency of migraine as a stroke preventative strategy. He was also started on ASA, and his medical risk factors were monitored. Furthermore, patients who are smokers or are taking oral contraception should be counseled on the risks of their continued use because both factors appear to have a major influence on stroke risk in this population. Although in migraineurs there is an association of stroke with the presence of a patent foramen ovale, there is no evidence that shunt closure reduces the risk of migraine-related stroke or frequency of migraine attacks. Last, certain vasoactive migraine abortifacients, such as triptans and ergot alkaloids, could theoretically cause reversible vasoconstriction and subsequent stroke. Such medications therefore may be considered contraindicated in a stroke population; however, there is increasing evidence that triptan use does not result in increased rates of stroke in patients with low cardiovascular risk.

- Migraine may be a risk factor for stroke, particularly in the posterior circulation. This risk is particularly high in patients who experience migraine aura or in those who are smokers or who take oral contraceptives.
- Migrainous stroke is a rare occurrence, and thorough evaluation of other etiologies is needed.
- Although there are no high-level clinical trial data, it is advised to control vascular risk factors and avoid medications that can potentially induce vasoconstriction in patients with migraine-related stroke.

Further Reading

Dowson A, Mullen MJ, Peatfield R, et al. Migraine intervention with STARFlex technology (MIST) trial. A prospective multicenter double-blind, sham-controlled trial to evaluate the effectiveness of patent foramen ovale closure with STARFlex septal repair implant to resolve refractory migraine headache. *Circulation* 2008;1117:1397–1404.

Etminan M, Takkouche B, Isorna FC, et al. Risk of ischaemic stroke in people with migraine: Systematic review and meta-analysis of observational studies. *BMJ* 2005;330:63.

Harriott AM, Barrett KM. Dissecting the association between migraine and stroke. *Curr Neurol Neurosci Rep* 2015;15(3):5.

Headache Classification Committee of the International Headache Society. The international classification of headache disorders, 3rd edition (beta version). *Cephalalgia* 2013;33(9):629–808.

Stang PE, Carson AP, Rose KM, et al. Headache, cerebrovascular symptoms, and stroke: The Atherosclerosis Risk in Communities Study. *Neurology* 2005;64:1573–1577.

Swartz RH, Kern RZ. Migraine is associated with magnetic resonance imaging white matter abnormalities. *Arch Neurol* 2004;61:1366–1368.

22 Driving Is a Headache

A 40-year-old man with no significant medical history developed altered mental status while driving a bus. He had been well until a week prior to admission, when he developed flu-like symptoms. He had nausea, vomiting, and a band-like headache. On the day of admission, he was driving a bus and felt unusual. He missed his turn and hit a pole. He does not remember anything after this. He was brought to the ER and was witnessed to be combative. He had a generalized tonic clonic seizure in the ER. A CT scan showed a right frontal ICH and a small right sylvian SAH. There was hyperdensity in the region of the right transverse sinus and superior sagittal sinus (Figure 22.1).

What do you do now?

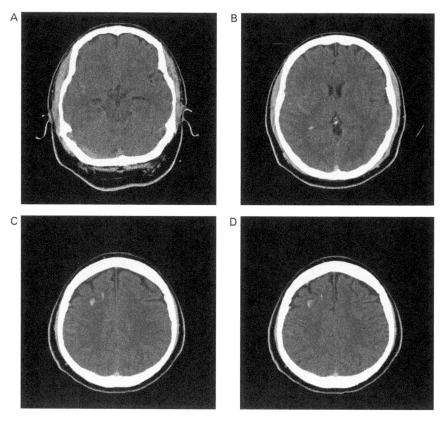

FIGURE 22.1 (A) CT showing hyperdensity along the right transverse sinus. (B) Right sylvian subarachnoid blood and hyperdensity in the superior saggital sinus. (C and D) Small hemorrhages in the right frontal lobe.

DURAL VENOUS SINUS THROMBOSIS

The findings on the noncontrast head CT are suggestive of dural venous sinus thrombosis. The hyperdensities in the area of the transverse sinus and superior saggital sinus strongly indicate this. He also has cortical hemorrhages that may be due to venous congestion.

Dural venous sinus thrombosis is a rare disease in which thrombosis of intracranial veins and/or sinuses occurs. Patients are younger (mean age in one series was 39 years) and more commonly female. The most common causes are prothrombotic state, such as hereditary thrombophilia, pregnancy or puerperium, and oral contraceptive use. Infections such as otitis or mastoiditis can cause local inflammation and thrombosis as well. This is more common in children. Head trauma and lumbar puncture have also been suggested as risk factors for venous thrombosis.

Patients most commonly present with headache, which is typically acute or subacute in onset. Patients may develop altered mental status, and seizures occur in 40% of patients. Imaging can show venous infarcts, often with hemorrhage. Initial CT findings may show hyperdensity in the region of the sinus (as in this patient), and contrast studies may show an "empty delta" sign in which there is no contrast opacification of the confluence of sinuses. Diagnosis is usually confirmed by MR venography (MRV) or CT venography.

Treatment is usually with anticoagulation. Clinicians are often nervous about this because there is hemorrhage on CT. However, it must be kept in mind that the hemorrhage is due to venous thrombosis and back pressure from poor venous drainage. The treatment of the underlying thrombosis should reduce the risk of recurrent hemorrhage. There are no large randomized trial data to support this. However, in a large registry with more than 600 patients, 80% were treated with anticoagulation showing usual clinical practice. There was 8% mortality in this study, and risk factors for poor outcome included being male, age older than 37 years, coma, ICH, deep venous system involvement, and cancer.

This patient had an MRI and MRV that confirmed dural venous sinus thrombosis. He was placed on low-molecular-weight heparin and transitioned to warfarin. He was also placed on leviteracetam for seizures. He recovered fully. He had a full hypercoagulable evaluation, which revealed a homozygous mutation of MTHFR C677. He continued warfarin for a year and then was switched to ASA. He remained symptom free and without recurrent thrombosis.

KEY POINTS TO REMEMBER

· Headache and hemorrhagic infarcts in patients who are hypercoagulable (including pregnancy and puerperium) should prompt an evaluation for dural venous sinus thrombosis.
· Treatment is typically with anticoagulation, despite hemorrhage on imaging.

Further Reading
Ferro JM, Canhao P, Stam J, et al. Prognosis of cerebral vein and dural sinus thrombosis: Results of the International Study on Cerebral Vein and Dural Sinus Thrombosis (ISCVT). *Stroke* 2004;35:664–670.
Stam J. Thrombosis of the cerebral veins and sinuses. *N Engl J Med* 2005;352:1791–1798.

23 Puff of Smoke

A 43-year-old woman developed recurrent neurological events. She developed intermittent episodes of left face and arm tingling and clumsiness of the left hand. She also had dysarthria. These episodes were recurrent and lasted 1 hour. She was seen at another hospital and was found to have multiple infarcts in both hemispheres. She had an angiogram and was told she had vasculitis. She was treated with corticosteroids, which precipitated depression and mania requiring a psychiatric hospitalization. She was placed on multiple antipsychotic medications and subsequently transferred to you. On your examination, she is tangential and grandiose but otherwise neurologically nonfocal. Figures 23.1 and 23.2 show the results of her imaging.

What do I do now?

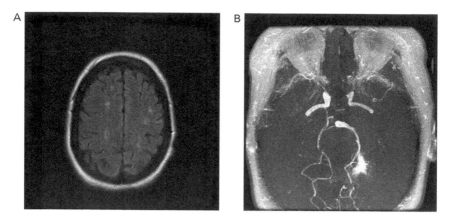

FIGURE 23.1 (A) MRI with bilateral chronic infarcts in a distal ICA territory. (B) MRA with occlusion of both ICAs.

MOYAMOYA DISEASE

This patient is having recurrent TIAs. Her pattern of infarcts on MRI is suggestive of distal ICA watershed infarcts. Her MRA shows bilateral distal ICA occlusions. This is confirmed by conventional cerebral angiography. In a young patient with bilateral ICA occlusive disease, moyamoya disease (MMD) should be considered. This type of occlusive disease is not consistent with central nervous system vasculitis.

Moyamoya is a rare disease in which there is spontaneous, progressive bilateral stenosis or occlusion of the terminal portion of the ICAs and their proximal branches in the circle of Willis. An abnormal vascular network of collateral blood vessels develops at the base of the brain that has an angiographic appearance of a

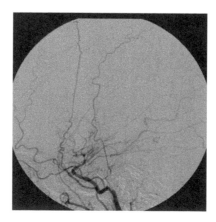

FIGURE 23.2 Cerebral angiogram showing occlusion of the ICA and prominent lenticulostriate vessels.

"puff of smoke," which is interpreted as "moyamoya" in Japanese. Pathologically, the affected intracranial arteries appear to develop intimal thickening with smooth muscle proliferation and often luminal thrombosis. The dilated collaterals demonstrate evidence of hemodynamic stress on the vessel wall, including fragmented elastic lamina, thinned media, and microaneurysm formation. MRI studies have shown outer-diameter narrowing of the affected vessels, suggesting vasoconstrictive changes not typical of atherosclerosis.

Although 10 times more prevalent in Asian populations, MMD can be seen in various race/ethnic groups. The prevalence of the disease, ranging from 3 to 10 per 100,000 persons in Asian countries, has been increasing in recent years due to improvements in diagnostic imaging. In addition, there is nearly a 2:1 female predominance and a bimodal age distribution, with peak incidences during early childhood and in the mid-forties. Although MMD is currently considered an idiopathic process, there is likely a genetic component. Fifteen percent of patients in Japan are suspected to have a familial form of MMD, and recently a single mutation in *RNF213* was discovered to be the first susceptibility gene for MMD. A moyamoya-like vasculopathy, similar to that seen in moyamoya disease, has been associated with multiple other medical conditions in what is termed moyamoya syndrome (Box 23.1).

Patients may present with either ischemic stroke (as a result of progressive ICA stenosis) or hemorrhage (due to the hemodynamic stress placed on fragile, compensatory neocollaterals). Hemorrhage is more common in adults and Asian

---

BOX 23.1 **Clinical Conditions Associated with Moyamoya Syndrome**

More Common

Cranial radiation
Sickle cell disease
Neurofibromatosis type 1
Down's syndrome
Graves' disease
Intracranial atherosclerosis
Head trauma

Less Common

Congenital cardiac anomaly
Lupus anticoagulant
Turner syndrome
Noonan syndrome
Fibromuscular dysplasia

populations and is rare in children. Symptoms of the disease, such as headaches and seizures, can also occur. The natural history of MMD is quite poor. Almost two-thirds of patients have symptomatic progression within 5 years. The rate of recurrent bleeding is 7% per year, and even asymptomatic disease has a 3.2% annual stroke risk. However, surgical revascularization seems to improve outcome, particularly if the patient has good functional status on presentation.

Medically, patients are often treated with antiplatelet therapy to reduce the risk of stroke from thrombi formed at areas of stenosis. Anticoagulation is not used, especially because there is a risk of ICH from rupture of friable collateral vessels. However, it is unclear whether antithrombotic usage in patients with MMD affects outcomes, and patients who radiologically progress or have recurrent symptoms, despite medical therapy, will likely require surgery.

There are no clinical trials to assess different revascularization treatments in patients presenting with ischemic stroke or TIA. There appears to be benefit with surgical treatment in preventing ischemia and improving cerebral hemodynamics, functional outcomes, and symptoms of headache or cognitive dysfunction. Although the initial experience was largely with children, observational data have confirmed similar benefits in adults who suffer ischemic stroke. Because the disease is limited to intracranial vessels, the goal is to redirect external carotid artery branches to supply the ischemic brain. Direct bypass can be performed with a microsurgical anastomosis of the superficial temporal artery to the middle cerebral artery allowing diversion of extracranial blood to the intracranial circulation. This allows for more rapid restoration of blood flow. Indirect bypass with encephaloduroarteriosynangiosis (EDAS) allows for external carotid artery branches found in richly vascularized tissues such as the dura, pericranium, or temporalis muscle to develop collateral flow to the ischemic brain over time. Direct and indirect techniques may be combined as well. It is unclear which method is superior because no randomized comparisons have been made. The recently published Japan Adult Moyamoya (JAM) trial assessed the benefit of bilateral, direct bypass in 80 Japanese adults who presented with ICH. Although there was a small number of patients included in the trial, there was a marginally significant benefit of surgery on rates of rebleeding at 5 years. These results indicated that surgical revascularization not only influences cerebral perfusion but also has additional effects on neocollaterals by eliminating hemodynamic stress on these fragile vessels. The benefit on rebleeding risk demonstrated in the JAM trial was particularly pronounced in patients presenting with hemorrhage from posterior circulation collaterals, such as thalamoperforators or the posterior choroidal artery.

In this patient, hemodynamic studies confirmed failure of cerebral perfusion. She initially underwent a right-sided EDAS, followed 2 months later by left EDAS. She has had no recurrent strokes on follow-up.

KEY POINTS TO REMEMBER

· Moyamoya is a rare cause of stroke in the United States. It is more common in Asian populations, particularly in patients presenting with ICH.
· Angiographic findings of distal ICA stenosis with lenticulostriate or choroidal neocollaterals are important in the diagnosis of MMD.
· A similar pathophysiological state to MMD is associated with several clinical conditions, some of which are acquired and some of which have a genetic etiology.
· Treatment is with surgical revascularization, which can reduce both ischemic and hemorrhagic complications.

Further Reading

Guzman R, Lee M, Achrol A, et al. Clinical outcome after 450 revascularization procedures for moyamoya disease. *J Neurosurg* 2009;111:927–935.

Kronenburg A, Braun KP, van der Zwan A, et al. Recent advances in moyamoya disease: Pathophysiology and treatment. *Curr Neurol Neurosci Rep* 2014;14:423.

Miyamoto S, Yoshimoto T, Hashimoto N, et al. Effects of extracranial–intracranial bypass for patients with hemorrhagic moyamoya disease: Results of the Japan Adult Moyamoya Trial. *Stroke* 2014;45:1415–1421.

Scott RM, Smith ER. Moyamoya disease and moyamoya syndrome. *N Engl J Med* 2009;360:1226–1237.

24 Thunderclap Headache

A 46-year-old woman with only high cholesterol presented with the worst headache of her life while traveling in Asia. She developed acute holocephalic headache that radiated down into the neck. The headache was maximal in intensity at onset. She took two aspirins with minimal relief. She went to a local clinic and was found to have an SBP of 170. A head CT was reportedly normal, and she was given pain medications. She returned to the United States 3 days later and saw a neurologist, who sent her to the ER. She was neurologically normal. Her imaging showed a small amount of SAH on CT that was confirmed on MRI (Figure 24.1).

What do you do now?

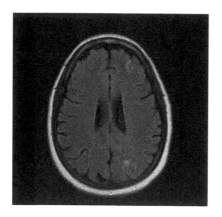
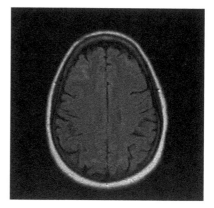

FIGURE 24.1   MRI FLAIR showing hyperintensities in sulci consistent with SAH.

REVERSIBLE CEREBRAL VASOCONSTRICTION SYNDROME

This presentation of thunderclap headache needs to be evaluated emergently for aneurysmal SAH. Her imaging, however, is not suggestive of aneurysmal hemorrhage because the distribution of blood is patchy and not in a typical location for a berry aneurysm rupture. An angiogram is warranted to evaluate for vascular anomalies. Her angiogram showed areas of focal stenoses (Figure 24.2).

This pattern of focal stenoses is highly suggestive of reversible cerebral vasoconstriction syndrome (RCVS). Historically, this disorder was called Call–Fleming syndrome, and early reports were in women during pregnancy or the puerperium. Migraines, medications such as selective serotonin reuptake inhibitors, and sympathomimetic drugs have also now been associated with the disorder. The diagnosis is based on clinical history and imaging findings. There are no

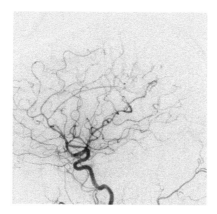

FIGURE 24.2   Cerebral angiogram showing focal stenoses primarily in the ACA branches.

serologic or CSF markers of the disease. The diagnosis is confirmed by spontaneous reversal of the angiographic abnormality.

In a case series of patients with RCVS, the authors found the disease was more common in a younger age group (mean age, 42 years) and in women. A total of 81% of RCVS patients have brain lesions on imaging, including ischemic stroke, convexity SAH, lobar ICH, and brain edema. Calcium channel blockers and glucocorticoids have been used in this disorder, but it is unclear if there is an effect on outcomes. The prognosis is typically good.

This patient had a very benign course, with resolution of headaches. She was placed on verapamil, a calcium channel blocker. She had a follow-up angiogram 4 weeks later that showed reversal of vasoconstriction.

KEY POINTS TO REMEMBER

- Severe thunderclap headaches warrant an immediate evaluation for SAH.
- Reversible vasoconstriction syndrome is associated with pregnancy and puerperium but may occur spontaneously or in association with medications or migraine.
- Empiric steroids and calcium channel blockers have been used, but there are no data to support this.

Further Reading

Singhal AB, Hajj-Ali RA, Topcuoglu MA, et al. Reversible cerebral vasoconstriction syndromes: Analysis of 139 cases. *Arch Neurol* 2011;68(8):1005–1012.

25 Hypertension and Confusion

An 83-year-old woman with hypertension, high cholesterol, and large cell lung cancer in remission was found by her son in the morning unresponsive and exhibiting shaking movements of her right arm and leg. She had been normal when she went to bed the night before. She was brought to the ER, and her abnormal movements stopped. Her blood pressure was 180/110. She was lethargic. She had no spontaneous movements in her arms or legs. She did not blink to threat in either visual field. She withdrew her arms and legs to deep stimulation.

What do you do now?

POSTERIOR REVERSIBLE ENCEPHALOPATHY SYNDROME

This is a patient with acute encephalopathy and seizure with an elevated blood pressure. Although encephalopathic, lack of blinking to threat on examination indicates possible vision loss. These clinical findings should raise suspicion for posterior reversible encephalopathy syndrome (PRES). There are many other toxic, infectious, or alternative vascular etiologies to consider in a patient with such a presentation. Given her prior history of lung cancer and new-onset focal seizure, metastatic disease should also be considered. An MRI was done to evaluate further.

Her MRI (Figure 25.1) showed symmetric posterior white matter change that was consistent with PRES. PRES is a clinical–radiographic syndrome of progressive headaches, blurred vision, confusion, and seizures in the setting of vasogenic edema on brain imaging, which is often localized to the posterior white matter. PRES is a disorder with unclear pathophysiology. A possible mechanism is that elevated blood pressure, hormonal changes, or toxic exposures in the setting of poor autoregulation of cerebral blood vessels leads to endothelial dysfunction and break down of the blood–brain barrier causing edema. This vasogenic edema can be detected on CT, but MRI has greater sensitivity.

MRI typically shows bilateral vasogenic edema in the parietal/occipital lobes, hence the description of the syndrome as a posterior encephalopathy. The posterior circulation may be more susceptible to autoregulatory failure. However, abnormal edema may also be present in other patterns: anterior, watershed, and within the basal ganglia or posterior fossa. Restricted diffusion, indicating infarction, can also be seen. Intracerebral hemorrhage can occur in 15% of cases, also presumably due to elevated blood pressure and poor cerebral autoregulation. Follow-up imaging in most cases shows reversal of edema, but resolution of the disease may take weeks.

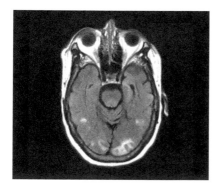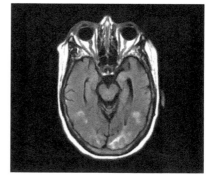

FIGURE 25.1 MRI demonstrating vasogenic edema within the white matter of the temporal and occipital lobes consistent with PRES.

PRES can be a difficult diagnosis to make. There are no specific diagnostic criteria or guidelines for evaluation and treatment. Risk factors for developing PRES are myriad and include fluctuating blood pressure, autoimmune disorders, certain chemotherapeutic drugs, immunosuppressants, sepsis, renal failure, and preeclampsia (Box 25.1). Clinically, patients can have headache, vision change (vision loss, cortical blindness, or hemianopia), encephalopathy, seizures, and even focal neurological deficits. Because these findings can be nonspecific, imaging, especially MRI, is necessary. Clinical features and imaging findings, particularly reversal of the abnormalities, support the diagnosis, but there is no pathognomonic finding.

Treatment is to remove the inciting agent. If elevated blood pressure is presumed to be the cause, the blood pressure is treated. Medications associated with PRES are stopped. In patients with eclampsia/preeclampsia with PRES,

---

BOX 25.1 **Risk Factors/Exposures Associated with PRES**

Chemotherapeutic and immunosuppressive agents
  Cisplatin, carboplatin, cytarabine, methotrexate, vincristine,
  l-asparaginase
  Bevacizumab
  Rituximab, infliximab, etanercept
  Cyclosporine, tacrolimus, sirolimus
  High-dose corticosteroid therapy
Hypertensive encephalopathy
Sepsis
  Most commonly gram-positive organisms
Preeclampsia or eclampsia
Autoimmune disease (common overlap with immunosuppressive
  agents)
  Systemic lupus erythematosus and/or anti-phospholipid
    antibody syndrome
  Scleroderma
  Polyarteritis nodosa
  Wegener's granulomatosis
  Rheumatoid arthritis
  Sjögren's syndrome
  Hashimoto's thyroiditis
  Thrombotic thrombocytopenic purpura
Renal failure
Sympathetic surge
  Pheochromocytoma, Cushing's syndrome
  Cocaine and amphetamine use

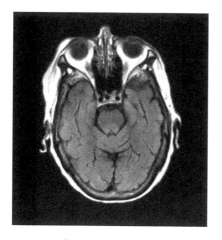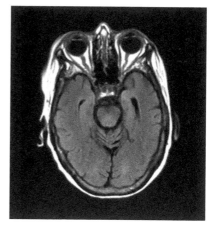

FIGURE 25.2 Repeat MRI 8 weeks later showing resolution of edema following blood pressure control.

magnesium sulfate is typically used first to treat both seizures and high blood pressure, with additional antihypertensives or anticonvulsants administered as needed.

This patient was treated with intravenous blood pressure medication to rapidly treat the blood pressure. There are no guidelines for the type of antihypertensive medication or goal blood pressure. She was treated with an intravenous calcium channel blocker with a goal to decrease her blood pressure initially by 25% in the first 24 hours, similar to treatment of malignant hypertension with any end organ damage. Recent data have shown that subsequent stroke rates following a diagnosis of hypertensive encephalopathy are equivalent or even higher than those observed following TIA. Therefore, careful follow-up and long-term blood pressure control should be instituted in patients with PRES due to hypertensive disease.

Her neurologic function improved with blood pressure control. She had follow-up imaging with an MRI 8 weeks later, which showed resolution of edema (Figure 25.2).

KEY POINTS TO REMEMBER

· Suspect PRES in patients presenting with hypertension and clinical symptoms of headache, mental status change, visual disturbance, or seizure.

· Other exposures associated with PRES include a clinical history of immunosuppressive or chemotherapeutic agent exposure, drug use,

systemic autoimmune disease, pregnancy and the puerperium, renal failure, and sepsis.
- Brain imaging often shows reversible, bilateral vasogenic edema in the posterior white matter regions and is necessary to rule out other etiologies or document concurrent infarction or hemorrhage.
- The treatment is not standardized and involves removing the offending agent and controlling blood pressure.

Further Reading

Bartynski WS. Posterior reversible encephalopathy syndrome: Part 1. Fundamental imaging and clinical features. *Am J Neuroradiol* 2008;29:1036–1042.

Cozzolino M, Bianchi C, Mariani G, et al. Therapy and differential diagnosis of posterior reversible encephalopathy syndrome (PRES) during pregnancy and postpartum. *Arch Gynecol Obstet* 2015;292:1217–1223.

Fugate JE, Rabinstein AA. Posterior reversible encephalopathy syndrome: Clinical and radiological manifestations, pathophysiology, and outstanding questions. *Lancet Neurol* 2015;14:914–925.

Lerario MP, Merkler AE, Gialdini G, et al. Risk of stroke after the International Classification of Diseases–Ninth Revision discharge code diagnosis of hypertensive encephalopathy. *Stroke* 2016;47(2):372–375.

26 A Protean Presentation

A 67-year-old man with hypertension is readmitted to the hospital with a stepwise progressive neurological decline over several months and worsening headache. His symptoms involve a worsening of his previous slurred speech, left facial droop, visual field cut, and new clumsiness of his left arm. A brain MRI from 1 month ago found hemorrhagic subacute infarcts of the right frontal operculum and right parietal–occipital regions with surrounding vasogenic edema (Figure 26.1). A laboratory workup was unremarkable, and his blood cultures and ESR were normal. The patient was negative for HIV, with normal rheumatological and hypercoagulable serological screens. MRA showed no significant stenosis. Cardiac workup was unremarkable, including TEE and extended telemetry. A lumbar puncture was notable for elevated protein, with negative CSF cytology and infectious studies. He has been treated with aspirin and statin for suspected cryptogenic embolic infarcts.

What do you do now?

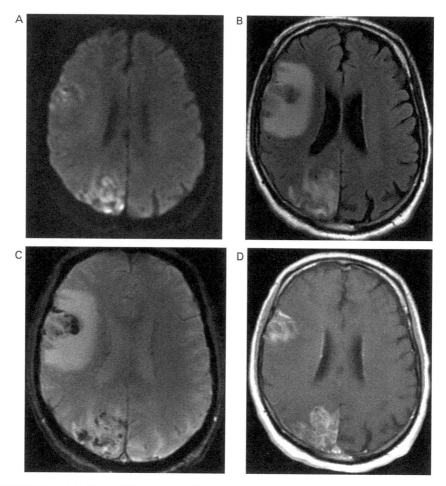

FIGURE 26.1 Initial brain MRI showing right frontal and right parieto-occipital subacute infarcts with associated hemorrhage and surrounding vasogenic edema causing mild local mass effect. MRI sequences are DWI (A), FLAIR (B), susceptibility-weighted imaging (C), and T1 post-contrast (D).

PRIMARY ANGIITIS OF THE CENTRAL NERVOUS SYSTEM

Despite an initially thorough stroke workup, this patient is still without a definitive diagnosis and continues to clinically progress. The differential diagnosis for a patient with this presentation and MRI findings is quite broad and includes vascular, neoplastic, inflammatory, and infectious causes. However, in a patient with multifocal, otherwise-unexplained lesions—particularly if they are hemorrhagic and/or mass-like—a vasculitic etiology should be considered.

Primary central nervous system (CNS) angiitis is a notably rare disorder with an estimated 2.4 cases per 1 million person-years. The disease involves inflammation of small and medium-sized leptomeningeal and parenchymal arteries within the CNS, without evidence of systemic involvement. The presentation can be highly variable in terms of the acuity of onset, location of CNS involvement, clinical symptomatology, and imaging characteristics. The clinical presentation can be acute, subacute, chronic, or recurrent with relapses and remissions. Any part of the CNS may be involved, including the brain (gray or white matter), spine, and optic nerves; multiple vascular territories are affected in up to 50% of cases. As would be expected from the unpredictable location of CNS involvement, clinical symptoms can be protean (Box 26.1). Imaging studies may demonstrate diverse-appearing lesions that range from ischemic to hemorrhagic (or both). In addition, enhancing and mass-like lesions, vessel wall and leptomeningeal enhancement, and confluent white matter disease have all been reported.

The wide variety of clinical presentations within the same disease entity makes standardized diagnostic criteria difficult. However, some proposed criteria include an acquired neurological deficit that remains unexplained after a thorough investigation, without evidence of a systemic vasculitis, and either classic angiographic or histopathologic features of vasculitis within the CNS. Nevertheless, making a diagnosis of primary CNS angiitis remains a clinical challenge (Box 26.2). Each patient who presents with stroke and suspected vasculitis should have a thorough stroke workup to rule out large artery or cardioembolic causes of infarction. In addition, inflammatory and infectious diseases should be evaluated for, and testing for ESR, C-reactive protein (CRP), rheumatologic markers such as antinuclear antibody

BOX 26.2   **Recommended Diagnostic Evaluation for Primary CNS Angiitis**

Serum: ESR, CRP, ANA, ANCA; screening for Lyme disease, HIV, syphilis
Imaging: Brain MRI, noninvasive angiography of the head and neck
Cardiac: Thorough echocardiography and telemetry monitoring
Lumbar puncture
Diagnostic cerebral angiogram
Brain biopsy

(ANA) and anti-neutrophil cytoplasmic antibody (ANCA), Lyme disease, HIV, and syphilis should not be indicative that the patient's CNS manifestations are secondary to another systemic disease process. Lumbar puncture is abnormal in approximately 90% of biopsy-proven cases, with typically mild to moderate elevations in protein levels and/or white blood cell counts. Angiography evaluating for alternating arterial stenoses and dilatations has been known to have a notoriously low sensitivity (42%) and positive predictive value (19%) when performed on biopsy-proven cases of primary CNS angiitis. The gold standard for diagnosis is a cortical and leptomeningeal biopsy demonstrating vessel wall inflammation. Biopsy for detecting vasculitis has been shown to have a sensitivity up to 63% in one series; however, other authors have reported much higher rates of false-negative biopsy results. Regardless, even if the biopsy does not rule in vasculitis as the diagnosis, the pathological evaluation may help determine an alternative diagnosis (a vasculitis mimic), such as demyelinating, infectious, or neoplastic diseases.

Although primary CNS angiitis may result in a high mortality if left untreated, patients seem to be relatively responsive to corticosteroids. The survival rate in more recent, treated patient cohorts is 85% at 1 year and 65% at 10 years. The mainstay of acute treatment is corticosteroid therapy, with or without cyclophosphamide, depending on the aggressiveness of the initial disease course. Such a treatment method has an 80–85% rate of achieving remission, although one-fourth of patients will eventually have a relapse. Azathioprine or mycophenolate mofetil can be used as steroid-sparing agents for maintenance therapy in patients who do have an initial response. Because of the rarity of the disease process, there are no randomized trials evaluating the treatment of primary CNS angiitis.

This patient underwent cerebral angiography, which was unremarkable, and he required two separate biopsies prior to obtaining a definite histological confirmation of a CNS vasculitis diagnosis (Figure 26.2). Prior to the second biopsy

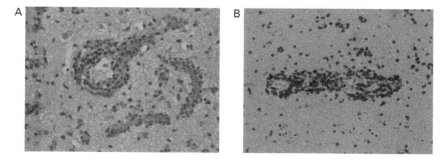

FIGURE 26.2 Pathology from right frontal brain biopsy demonstrating T cell lymphocytic-type primary angiitis of the CNS. (A) Hematoxylin and eosin stain; (B) CD3 immunohistochemical stain.

returning positive results, the patient was again readmitted to the hospital with progressive neurological decline and had an increase in the size and enhancement of his cerebral lesions. He was empirically started on corticosteroids and cyclophosphamide.

KEY POINTS TO REMEMBER

· Primary CNS angiitis can present with variable clinical symptoms, location of CNS involvement, and imaging characteristics.
· Consider a diagnosis of vasculitis in patients with atypical-appearing or multifocal vascular lesions, particularly if they involve both ischemic and hemorrhagic components.
· It is imperative to first rule out the more common causes of stroke and systemic inflammatory diseases prior to entertaining a diagnosis of primary CNS angiitis.
· Often, a combination of both a cerebral angiogram and brain biopsy is required to obtain the diagnosis, although both have high rates of false-negative results.
· The disease is highly fatal if left untreated, but corticosteroids have greatly increased survival. If the disease is still suspected despite an inability to histopathologically confirm the diagnosis, empiric treatment should be considered, particularly if no other diagnosis is more likely after a thorough evaluation.

Further Reading

Calabrese LH, Mallek JA. Primary angiitis of the central nervous system: Report of 8 new cases, review of the literature, and proposal for diagnostic criteria. *Medicine (Baltimore)* 1988;67(1):20–39.

Miller DV, Salvarani C, Hunder GG, et al. Biopsy findings in primary angiitis of the central nervous system. *Am J Surg Pathol* 2009;33(1):35–43.

Powers J. Primary angiitis of the central nervous system diagnostic criteria. *Neurol Clin* 2015;33:515–526.

Salvarini C, Brown RD, Christianson T, et al. An update of the Mayo Clinic cohort of patients with adult primary central nervous system vasculitis. *Medicine* 2015;94(21):1–15.

27 Can I Go Home Now?

A 56-year-old man with a history of metastatic prostate cancer and tobacco abuse presented with two episodes of right-sided weakness. He developed acute numbness and weakness on the right and was unable to talk. He fell because of the weakness. Symptoms lasted 10 minutes and resolved completely. One hour later, he had recurrence of the same symptoms and again resolved. He came to the ER and was found to have a normal examination. His blood pressure was 120/88. His CT was normal. He is unable to get an MRI because of metal in his body. The patient would like to go home.

What do you do now?

TRANSIENT ISCHEMIC ATTACK DIAGNOSIS AND MANAGEMENT

This patient has presented with a TIA. He had acute-onset, self-resolving neurological symptoms referable to a known vascular territory: In this case, he experienced a brief, left middle cerebral artery syndrome consisting of right hemiparesis and aphasia. The clinical and research definition of TIA has been evolving to include a shorter, more-defined time period, as well as the use of imaging studies. The traditional definition was time-based, with the neurological symptoms expected to have resolved within 24 hours. This 24-hour time limit was arbitrary. The majority of TIA patients have symptoms lasting less than 1 hour, and only 14% have symptoms lasting more than 6 hours. In addition, the older definition does not fit with the timing of irreversible brain infarction, which can be found on MRI in one-third to one-half of patients with symptoms less than 24 hours. The more recently proposed definition of TIA includes a shorter duration of symptoms and imaging as a marker of permanent tissue injury, with the intent to more clearly delineate transient, reversible ischemia (i.e., TIA) from completed infarction (i.e., stroke). This definition of TIA is as follows: symptoms typically less than 1 hour and without evidence of infarct on imaging.

There have been attempts at risk stratification of TIA patients. The $ABCD_2$ score is commonly used (Box 27.1).

This scale may help identify patients who are at high risk of early recurrence or subsequent stroke. In one study, the risk of recurrent stroke or TIA was 8% at 48 hours in patients with the highest $ABCD_2$ scores. However, other studies have found that the $ABCD_2$ score may overestimate the subsequent risk of stroke, and its ability to clinically predict recurrence is poor if utilized by non-neurologists. Observational studies have previously shown that the $ABCD_2$ system can be used safely to help triage patients for expedited inpatient workup, as opposed to outpatient follow-up, and reduce hospitalizations. However, this use of the ABC_2 score may be falling out of favor because a recent meta-analysis

---

BOX 27.1   **$ABCD_2$ score**

A   Age >60 years: 1 point
B   Blood pressure >140/90: 1 point
C   Clinical features—weakness: 2 points; speech disturbance without weakness: 1 point; other: 0 points
D   Diabetes: 1 point
D_2 Duration—>60 minutes: 2 points; 10–59 minutes: 1 point; <10 minutes: 0 points

---

demonstrated it may not be able to confidently discriminate a true vascular event from a stroke mimic. Alternatively, 20% of patients classified as low-risk by the $ABCD_2$ system were actually found to have underlying high-risk mechanisms, such as atrial fibrillation or significant carotid stenosis, which may result in management changes. Therefore, imaging studies, particularly non-invasive angiography and brain MRI, may also be of use in triaging potential TIA patients presenting to the emergency department. Studies have suggested that patients who have evidence of acute infarct on MRI, despite clinical resolution of symptoms, are at particularly high risk of recurrence. Nonetheless, no randomized trials exist to test the ability of the $ABCD_2$ score to triage patients effectively.

Regardless of $ABCD_2$ score, we generally admit all patients with true TIA to expedite a workup. Workup should include brain imaging, vascular imaging, and cardiac evaluation with at least an ECG and an echocardiogram. Hospitalization is usually the quickest way to complete an evaluation and start a prevention program. However, other means of rapid evaluation and treatment, such as a TIA clinic, have been shown to improve outcomes. Introduction of more urgent stroke assessment and treatment in a specialized clinic has been associated with an 80% reduction in the risk of early recurrent stroke.

Stroke prevention strategies in patients with TIA are similar to those in patients with ischemic stroke. Appropriate antithrombotic selection, statin usage, and aggressive risk factor management are key components of an effective secondary stroke prevention regimen. In the CHANCE trial, patients with minor ischemic stroke or high-risk TIA (defined as having an $ABCD_2$ score of 4 or greater) benefited from short-term dual antiplatelet agents compared to those treated with aspirin alone, without an increase in bleeding risk. In the SPARCL trial, patients with recent stroke or TIA, and no history of coronary artery disease, benefited from 80 mg of atorvastatin compared to placebo.

This patient was hospitalized for an evaluation that included an echocardiogram and vascular imaging. He was found to have a left middle cerebral artery stenosis and was treated with antiplatelets and statin. This patient's $ABCD_2$ score is 2 (1 point for weakness and 1 point for duration of symptoms). This case illustrates the failure of the $ABCD_2$ score to predict a high-risk arterial lesion. Had this patient not been hospitalized and undergone urgent noninvasive angiography, an intracranial stenosis would not have been discovered, a finding that would possibly change blood pressure management and antiplatelet agent selection.

Further Reading

Albers GW, Caplan LR, Easton JD, et al. Transient ischemic attack: Proposal for a new definition. *N Engl J Med* 2002;347:1713–1716.

Easton JD, Saver JL, Albers GW, et al. Definition and evaluation of transient ischemic attack: A scientific statement for healthcare professionals from the American Heart Association/American Stroke Association Stroke Council; Council on Cardiovascular Surgery and Anesthesia; Council on Cardiovascular Radiology and Intervention; Council on Cardiovascular Nursing; and the Interdisciplinary Council on Peripheral Vascular Disease. *Stroke* 2009;40:2276–2293.

Johnston SC, Rothwell PM, Nguyen-Huynh MN, et al. Validation and refinement of scores to predict very early stroke risk after transient ischaemic attack. *Lancet* 2007;369:283–292.

Olivot JM, Wolford C, Castle J, et al. TWO ACES: Transient ischemic attack work-up as outpatient assessment of clinical evaluation and safety. *Stroke* 2011;42:1839–1843.

Prabhakaran S, Chong JY, Saccco RL. Impact of abnormal diffusion-weighted imaging results on short-term outcome following transient ischemic attack. *JAMA Neurol* 2007;64(8):1105–1109.

Rothwell PM, Giles MF, Chandratheva A, et al. Effect of urgent treatment of transient ischaemic attack and minor stroke on early recurrent stroke (EXPRESS study): A prospective population based sequential comparison. *Lancet* 2007;370:1432–1442.

Wardlaw JM, Brazzelli M, Chappell FM, et al. $ABCD_2$ score and secondary stroke prevention: Meta-analysis and effect per 1000 patients triaged. *Neurology* 2015;85(4):373–380.

28 Cardiac Arrest

A 58-year-old man was witnessed to collapse at work. He was pulseless and unresponsive. A bystander immediately called emergency medical services (EMS) and started CPR. When EMS arrived, his cardiac rhythm was ventricular fibrillation. He was intubated and defibrillated in the field with return of spontaneous circulation in 10 minutes. He was brought to the ER, where he was initially moving all limbs and localized to pain. He was then placed on sedation. He had a bedside echocardiogram that showed a dilated and hypokinetic left ventricle. He had a cardiac catheterization and subsequent stenting of the left anterior descending artery. After the procedure, his intravenous sedation was stopped to reassess his neurological status, and he was found to be unresponsive with no movements in his arms or legs to noxious stimuli.

What do you do now?

ANOXIC BRAIN INJURY

This patient had a witnessed out-of-hospital cardiac arrest. He was rapidly resuscitated, but after the cardiac interventions, he was comatose and with no purposeful movements.

With cardiac arrest, there is interruption of cerebral blood flow causing global hypoxic–ischemic insult to the brain. The goal post-arrest is to try to minimize the degree of this damage. One means of mitigating the hypoxic insult is by instituting therapeutic hypothermia. Hypothermia has been considered neuroprotective, theoretically by decreasing the brain's metabolic demand.

Two randomized trials support the use of therapeutic hypothermia after cardiac arrest. A large study in Europe of patients with ventricular fibrillation (VF) and pulseless ventricular tachycardia (VT) arrest found a significant improvement in outcome in patients treated with hypothermia to 32–34°C for 24 hours compared to patients maintained at normothermia. A total of 55% of patient treated with hypothermia versus 39% of normothermic patients had favorable 6-month neurological outcome. Furthermore, patients treated with hypothermia had lower mortality and similar rates of complications. However, the normothermic patients in this trial had a mean temperature of 37.8°C, which could potentially exaggerate results when comparing them to those of patients in the hypothermic arm. The other trial randomized patients to 33°C or 37°C for 12 hours and also showed better outcomes based on discharge disposition in patients treated with hypothermia. In these studies, cooling was achieved within 2–4 hours of the return of spontaneous circulation, indicating that hypothermia should be initiated as soon as possible in comatose survivors of out-of-hospital arrest. These trials led to recommendations by different organizations to treat with therapeutic hypothermia for out-of-hospital cardiac arrest with VF or pulseless VT. Based on these trials, the American Heart Association recommends a target temperature of 32–34°C for 12–24 hours in comatose patients.

Recently, a large randomized trial compared a target temperature of 33°C versus 36°C. This trial randomized more than 900 patients. It found no significant difference between the groups in terms of death and poor neurological function at 6 months. This trial suggests a benefit of hypothermia with less aggressive temperature goals.

This patient had ventricular fibrillation arrest and coma. He was started on a therapeutic hypothermia protocol (Figure 28.1). Care should be taken to prevent shivering when inducing and maintaining hypothermia because this is a physiological response to combat lower body temperatures and may make it difficult

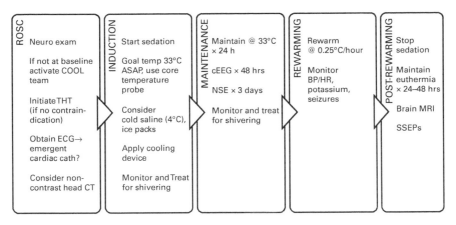

FIGURE 28.1 Suggested therapeutic hypothermia protocol.

to achieve the desired temperature ranges that result in neurological recovery. Various agents may be used to treat shivering, and depending on the severity of shivering response, these treatments range from acetaminophen, intravenous magnesium sulfate, skin counterwarming, and buspirone to opioid analgesics, sedatives, and neuromuscular paralytics in refractory cases.

After rewarming is an appropriate time to reassess the patient's examination to determine neurologic prognosis. Many factors may help guide prognostication.

Prognosis is typically based on the neurological exam at 24–72 hours after cardiac arrest. Findings that predict poor outcome include myoclonic status epilepticus and poor brainstem function. Poor brainstem function, especially the absence of pupillary response, absent corneals, and absent or extensor motor responses, is associated with poor outcomes.

Ancillary neurophysiological testing with EEG and somatosensory evoked potentials (SSEPs) are often performed. Abnormal findings on EEG such as burst suppression and absent N20 response on SSEP portend poor outcomes. SSEPs are performed in centers with trained technicians after the rewarming phase because hypothermia may affect the results. High serum neuron-specific enolase (NSE) levels (>33) are also associated with poor outcome, with low rates of false-positive test results. Typically, NSE levels are drawn during the first several days post-arrest until the values peak.

At 72 hours, this patient opened eyes to voice and tracked. He had normal pupils, eye movements, and corneal reflexes. He briskly withdrew his arms and legs to noxious stimuli. His NSE on day 3 was 11. His EEG showed rare left temporal sharp waves but no seizures. His SSEP with median nerve stimulation showed a response at the upper limit of normal. All of these findings were consistent with a good prognosis. Six months after his cardiac arrest, he was neurologically normal.

KEY POINTS TO REMEMBER

· Following cardiac arrest, therapeutic hypothermia should be initiated as soon as possible in comatose survivors, which improves discharge disposition and neurological outcomes at 6 months.

· Current guidelines recommend a goal temperature of 32–34°C maintained for 12–24 hours; however, recent data indicate that milder hypothermia targets may result in similar outcomes.

· Shivering in response to the hypothermia is common and should be treated aggressively.

· The neurological examination, as well as ancillary tests such as EEG monitoring, SSEP studies, and serum NSE levels, may collectively aid in the determination of neurological prognosis post-arrest.

Further Reading

Bernard SA, Gray TW, Buist MD, et al. Treatment of comatose survivors of out of hospital cardiac arrest with induced hypothermia. *N Engl J Med* 2002;346:557–563.

The Hypothermia after Cardiac Arrest Study Group. Mild therapeutic hypothermia to improve the neurologic outcome after cardiac arrest. *N Engl J Med* 2002;346:549–556.

Nielsen N, Wetterslev J, Cronberg T, et al. Targeted temperature management at 33°C versus 36°C after cardiac arrest. *N Engl J Med* 2013;369:2197–2206.

Peberdy MA, Callaway CW, Neumar RW, et al. Post cardiac arrest care: 2010 American Heart Association guidelines for cardiopulmonary resuscitation and emergency cardiovascular care. *Circulation* 2010;122:S768–S786.

Wijdicks EF, Hijdra A, Young GB, et al. Practice parameter: Prediction of outcome in comatose survivors after cardiopulmonary resuscitation (an evidence-based review): Report of the Quality Standards Subcommittee of the American Academy of Neurology. *Neurology* 2006;67:203–210.

29 A Sickle Pickle

A 13-year-old girl with a history of sickle cell disease
arrived in the ER with shortness of breath and right-sided
weakness. She had been having shortness of breath for a
day. She awoke the day of admission with right arm and
leg weakness and numbness. She also had some mild
headache. She had no change in speech. On examination,
she had no fever. Her heart rate was 128 and oxygen
saturation was 88% on room air. She had weakness in the
right arm and leg. Her MRI showed small scattered acute
infarcts in the left hemisphere (Figure 29.1) and chronic
right-sided infarcts. Her MRA showed distal left ICA and
proximal MCA stenoses (Figure 29.2).

What do you do now?

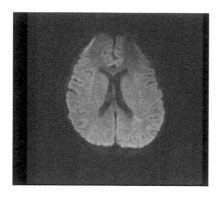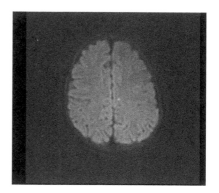

FIGURE 29.1 DWI sequence showing small acute infarctions in the left hemispheric watershed zones.

SICKLE CELL DISEASE AND STROKE

Sickle cell disease is an inherited hemoglobinopathy in which sickle cells cause vaso-occlusive disease affecting many organ systems. It can affect cerebral vessels and result in stroke. Stroke should be considered in children with sickle cell disease and acute neurologic deficit. Sickle cell disease is a potent risk factor for stroke in children. Children with sickle cell disease have more than a 200-fold increased risk of stroke compared with children without sickle cell disease. Approximately 11% of children with sickle cell disease will have a stroke by age 20 years, with the highest risk during the first decade of life. Predictors of clinical stroke include history of TIA, acute chest syndrome within the previous 2 weeks, degree of anemia, and elevated blood pressure. Increased velocity on transcranial Dopplers (TCDs) is also a significant risk factor for stroke.

The mechanism of stroke in patients with sickle cell disease is usually large vessel disease. Sickled cells can cause a large vessel arteriopathy, especially at the distal ICA, similar to that observed in moyamoya disease. The mechanism is

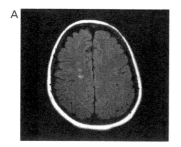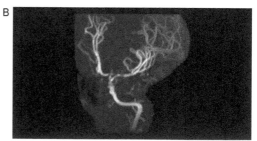

FIGURE 29.2 (A) FLAIR sequence showing linear scattered chronic infarcts in the right hemisphere. (B) MRA demonstrating intracranial stenosis of the distal ICA and proximal MCA.

thought to be due to intimal hyperplasia from chronic endothelial damage from sickled cells. Angiographic studies have found that a large proportion of patients with stroke also have large vessel stenoses as seen in this patient. Small vessel infarcts can also occur, and silent infarcts on imaging are more typically found in the white matter.

A stroke diagnosis in a patient with sickle cell disease is made with conventional imaging using either CT or MRI. TCD studies are a good screening tool for intracranial stenoses by evaluating for increased flow velocities in the distal ICA or other proximal vessels. MRA of the intracranial vessels can confirm large vessel stenosis.

The treatment of patients with sickle cell disease and stroke is primarily with exchange transfusion. Exchange transfusion provides normal red blood cells and improves blood flow with a lower proportion of sickled cells. The Stroke Prevention in Sickle Cell Anemia (STOP) trial showed that chronic exchange transfusions in children deemed high risk of stroke based on TCD velocities greater than 200 cm/sec significantly lowered the risk of stroke by more than 90%.

The STOP trial was a primary prevention trial, and because there are no secondary stroke prevention intervention trials for sickle cell disease, the results of STOP are used to support exchange transfusion after a clinical stroke and for prevention of recurrent stroke. Small studies of stopping transfusion therapy in patients who have had a stroke showed high risk of recurrent stroke after cessation. In one study, 5 of 10 patients had a recurrent stroke within 12 months of stopping treatment.

Unfortunately, there are long-term complications associated with chronic transfusion. Patients can develop infections and iron overload. A trial of hydroxyurea as an alternative to transfusion in children with stroke and iron overload randomized patients to determine noninferiority of hydroxyurea. This trial was stopped early after an interim analysis due to futility, and exchange transfusion remains the mainstay of treatment.

The American Heart Association recommends transfusions to reduce hemoglobin S to less than 30% of total hemoglobin. There are no data, especially in children, for the use of antiplatelets or statins for secondary stroke prevention in patients with sickle cell disease.

This girl with sickle cell disease had a stroke. Her clinical findings and imaging studies show acute stroke in the left hemisphere and chronic asymptomatic strokes in the right hemisphere. The infarct topography on the left is in the watershed territories between the MCA and anterior cerebral artery and the MCA and posterior cerebral artery. The right-sided infarcts are in a linear pattern seen in ICA borderzone infarcts. Both patterns suggest proximal large vessel disease with flow failure. During systemic stress such as infection, perfusion failure can occur and the watershed area is most vulnerable.

In the setting of acute stroke, it is important to maintain oxygenation, especially in the case of severe anemia. This patient was treated with supplemental oxygen. She had urgent exchange transfusion to lower the proportion of hemoglobin S. She was maintained on chronic exchange transfusion for secondary stroke prevention.

Although this patient awoke with stroke and therefore was out of the treatment window for IV thrombolysis, tPA administration in patients younger than age 18 years is controversial and largely unstudied. An international randomized trial, thrombolysis in pediatric stroke (TIPS), attempted to study the safety and efficacy of tPA in a pediatric population, but it was prematurely terminated after only 1 of 93 screened patients was enrolled. Retrospective, observational data from the Nationwide Inpatient Sample showed that 1.6% of pediatric stroke patients received tPA between 2000 and 2003. However, those patients who received tPA were less likely to be discharged home and had higher rates of death and dependency. The American Heart Association/American Stroke Association do not currently recommend the routine clinical treatment of pediatric stroke patients with IV tPA due to the unclear risks and benefits of thrombolysis in this population. Furthermore, sickle cell patients have high rates of intracranial hemorrhage at baseline, comprising almost one-third of cerebrovascular events. These patients may theoretically be at an increased risk of hemorrhagic complications with tPA administration.

KEY POINTS TO REMEMBER

- Patients with sickle cell disease should be screened for stroke risk using TCDs to evaluate for intracranial stenosis.
- Sickle cell patients with prior stroke or who have velocities >200 cm/sec on TCD studies should be treated with chronic exchange transfusions.
- Chronic exchange transfusions with a goal hemoglobin S fraction less than 30% should be continued indefinitely in patients with high risk for stroke.
- In patients with acute stroke, it is imperative to provide supplemental oxygenation as necessary.
- Intravenous thrombolysis for acute ischemic stroke is largely unstudied in pediatric populations and may be dangerous to

administer in sickle cell patients who have increased rates of
intracranial hemorrhage at baseline.

Further Reading

Adams RJ, McKie VC, Hsu L, et al. Prevention of a first stroke by transfusions in children
with sicle cell anemia and abnormal results on transcranial Doppler ultrasonography.
N Engl J Med 1998;339:5–11.

Janjua N, Nasar A, Lynch JK, et al. Thrombolysis for ischemic stroke in children: Data from
the Nationwide Inpatient Sample. *Stroke* 2007;38:1850–1854.

Rivkin MJ, de Veber G, Ichord RN, et al. Thrombolysis in pediatric stroke study. *Stroke*
2015;46:880–885.

Switzer JA, Hess DC, Fenwick TN, et al. Pathophysiology and treatment of stroke in sickle
cell disease: Present and future. *Lancet Neurol* 2006;5:501–512.

Wang WC, Kovnar EH, Tonkin IL, et al. High risk of recurrent stroke after discontinuance of
five to twelve years of transfusion therapy in patients with sickle cell disease.
J Pediatr 1991;118:377–382.

Ware, RE, Helms RW; SWiTCH Investigators. Stroke with transfusions changing to
hydroxyurea (SWiTCH). *Blood* 2012;26:3925–3932.

30 Numbness While on Anticoagulation

A 65-year-old woman with a history of hypertension and atrial fibrillation developed acute left leg numbness. She was on warfarin for atrial fibrillation but admits to poor compliance. She noticed numbness in the left foot when she was walking barefoot and did not feel the cold tiles as she felt with the right foot. She denied any headache, visual change, or motor symptoms. She saw her doctor, who requested an outpatient head CT. The CT revealed a hemorrhage, and she was sent to the ER. In the ER, her blood pressure was 205/78. She had mild weakness in the left arm and leg and dense sensory loss in the left leg. Her INR was normal. Her CT showed a hemorrhage in the right putamen (Figure 30.1).

What do you do now?

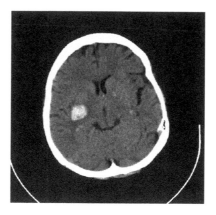

FIGURE 30.1 Head CT with hyperdensity in the right basal ganglia suggestive of hypertensive ICH.

HYPERTENSIVE INTRACEREBRAL HEMORRHAGE

Hemorrhagic stroke is associated with high morbidity and mortality, and patients with ICH are at risk for early clinical deterioration due to hematoma expansion. CT technology is readily accessible and allows for a rapid diagnosis in patients with ICH. The location and appearance of the hematoma in this patient are suggestive of hypertensive ICH. She has a history of hypertension and has a significantly elevated blood pressure on presentation. The typical locations for hypertensive hemorrhage include the basal ganglia, pons, cerebellum, and thalamus.

The immediate treatment should be to lower the blood pressure. Recent evidence suggests that aggressive, acute blood pressure reduction in the setting of ICH is safe and may improve clinical outcomes. The largest randomized trial evaluating the efficacy of intensive blood pressure lowering is the Intensive Blood Pressure Reduction in Acute Cerebral Hemorrhage Trial 2 (INTERACT2). This study assessed the effects of lowering systolic blood pressure to a goal of <140 mmHg within 1 hour of randomization in 2794 patients with acute ICH. There was a strong trend (p = 0.06) toward less death or major disability at 90 days in the intensive therapy group (52%) compared to those receiving standard blood pressure control (56%). Prespecified secondary analyses demonstrated significantly improved disability scores on the modified Rankin scale and better quality of life. There was no increase in death (12%) or serious adverse events (23%) observed in the intensive blood pressure-lowering group. An ongoing trial, Antihypertensive Treatment of Acute Cerebral Hemorrhage II (ATACH II), may confirm the findings observed in INTERACT2. The current American Heart Association guidelines for hypertensive hemorrhage recommend lowering systolic blood pressure to a target of 140/90. However, care should be taken in patients with large hematomas and elevated intracranial pressure (ICP) because abrupt declines in blood pressure may compromise cerebral perfusion in patients with increased ICP. In the INTERACT2 trial, the majority of ICH patients had small hematoma volumes (<20 mL), so the safety of aggressive blood pressure reduction in patients with larger hematomas is not as well-studied. In these situations, it is important to use a rapid-acting and easily titratable medication for blood pressure control. Intravenous drips such as nicardipine are often used.

The patient had been on warfarin but was noncompliant. In patients with coagulopathy and hemorrhage, coagulopathy should be corrected rapidly. In patients on warfarin, this may be done with IV vitamin K, fresh frozen plasma, or prothrombin complex concentrate (PCC). Emerging evidence suggests that PCCs may have fewer complications and correct the INR more rapidly than fresh frozen plasma. Patients taking direct thrombin or factor Xa inhibitors may also receive PCC, but reversal agents are currently on the market (idarucizumab) or in clinical trials (andexanet alfa). The benefit of platelet transfusions in patients on antiplatelet agents is unclear, but they are often administered, especially in patients with persistent bleeding. Anticonvulsants are not routinely recommended for prophylaxis unless there is high risk of seizures based on the hematoma characteristics or unless ICP is a concern (because seizure can increase ICP). Deep vein thrombosis prophylaxis is important in ICH patients because there are high rates of immobility. After 48 hours, if repeat imaging confirms that there is no hematoma expansion, subcutaneous heparin may be started for prophylaxis against venous thromboembolism.

Prevention of recurrent hemorrhage, especially in a patient with hypertensive hemorrhage, is to aggressively control blood pressure to normotension. Resumption of anticoagulation in patients with hemorrhage requires careful consideration of the risks and benefits. Anticoagulation in lobar ICH is usually not recommended because the likelihood of recurrent hemorrhage is higher with amyloid angiopathy. With small deep hemorrhages such as this, the risk of recurrent hemorrhage needs to be balanced against the risk of ischemic stroke from atrial fibrillation. Recent nonrandomized data suggest that rates of ischemic stroke following anticoagulant-associated ICH are notably high, and on a population level, patients may benefit from restarting anticoagulation without an increase in mortality or major hemorrhage. Further randomized trials are necessary to better evaluate the safety and efficacy of restarting anticoagulation in ICH patients, and the optimal time to resume antithrombotics has yet to be defined.

In this patient, anticoagulation was held for 3 months. Follow-up imaging showed resolution of the hematoma and blood pressure was well controlled. Her gradient echo sequence showed no evidence of other microhemorrhages on MRI that would indicate possible amyloid angiopathy. This patient was resumed on her warfarin for atrial fibrillation. Because the direct thrombin and factor Xa inhibitors have an overall reduced risk of ICH in patients with atrial fibrillation, it would be reasonable to have used one of these agents as an alternative to warfarin.

KEY POINTS TO REMEMBER

- Patients with suspected ICH should be immediately evaluated with CT scanning.
- If coagulopathic, correction of coagulopathy must be instituted rapidly.
- Blood pressure should be monitored and treated with a goal SBP of less than 140 when ICP is not elevated.
- In patients with atrial fibrillation and ICH, a careful analysis of each patient's risks and benefits must be performed prior to resuming anticoagulation for ischemic stroke prevention.

Further Reading

Anderson CS, Heeley E, Huang Y, et al.; for the INTERACT2 Investigators. Rapid blood-pressure lowering in patients with acute intracerebral hemorrhage. *N Engl J Med* 2013;368:2355–2365.

Hemphill JC, Greenberg SM, Anderson C, et al. Guidelines for the management of spontaneous intracerebral hemorrhage: A guideline for healthcare professionals from the American Heart Association/American Stroke Association. *Stroke* 2015;46.

Kuramatsu JB, Gerner ST, Schellinger PD, et al. Anticoagulant reversal, blood pressure levels, and anticoagulant resumption in patients with anticoagulation-related intracerebral hemorrhage. *JAMA* 2015;313(8):824–836.

Lerario MP, Gialdini G, Lapidus DM, et al. Risk of ischemic stroke after intracranial hemorrhage in patients with atrial fibrillation. *PLoS One* 2015;10(12):e0145579.

Nielsen PB, Larsen TB, Skjøth F, et al. Restarting anticoagulant treatment after intracranial hemorrhage in patients with atrial fibrillation and the impact on recurrent stroke, mortality, and bleeding: A nationwide cohort study. *Circulation* 2015;132(6):517–525.

31 Hemorrhage in a Patient with Dementia

A 69-year-old woman with prior intracerebral hemorrhages
and dementia presented with an acute decrease in verbal
output and somnolence. She had initially been seen
7 years prior to presentation with a right temporal ICH.
The hemorrhage was surgically evacuated, and pathology
revealed cerebral amyloid angiopathy. She had a right
frontal lobar hemorrhage 1 year after the first hemorrhage.
She remained stable and was ambulatory and conversant
but required 24-hour assistance because of cognitive
difficulty for the next few years. She now returns with
garbled speech. Her blood pressure was 177/72. She
was found to be awake and mumbling incoherently.
She did not follow any commands. She moved all
limbs spontaneously. A CT scan showed a new lobar
hemorrhage in the left Sylvian region (Figure 31.1).

What do you do now?

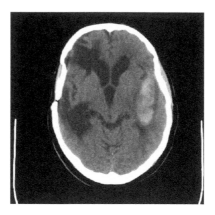

FIGURE 31.1   CT showing skull defect due to prior craniotomy, encephalomalacia in the right frontal and temporal lobes, and hyperdensity in the left temporal/insular lobes.

CEREBRAL AMYLOID ANGIOPATHY

Cerebral amyloid angiopathy (CAA) needs to be considered in a patient with multiple lobar hemorrhages. Lobar hemorrhage refers to the superficial location of blood products within a cortical or cortico-subcortical region. Such lobar bleeding tends to be multiple and recurrent in patients with CAA. This is in contrast to hypertensive hemorrhages, which classically occur in deep, subcortical or infratentorial areas. CAA is an important cause of ICH in the elderly because the prevalence of CAA increases with age. It is the second most common ICH etiology following hypertension.

CAA is caused by beta amyloid deposition in leptomeningeal and cortical vessels of the brain. This deposition can lead to small vessel occlusion and white matter disease. The vessels are also friable and may rupture causing hemorrhage, which can range from cortical microhemorrhages to lobar ICH and superficial siderosis (i.e., focal convexity subarachnoid hemorrhage). Cerebral microbleeds are more prevalent in patients with CAA and seem to occur at sites of increased amyloid deposition when correlated with amyloid positron emission tomography scans. Increasing burden of lobar microhemorrhages can predict the severity of CAA, as well as the future risk of ICH and mortality. Because of the pathological overlap with parenchymal amyloid deposition observed in Alzheimer's disease, there is a strong association of CAA with dementia. Furthermore, ApoE genotype has been linked to the risk of development of CAA, recurrent hemorrhages, and dementia.

The definitive diagnosis of CAA can only be made pathologically. The Boston Criteria have been developed to better categorize definite, probable, and possible

TABLE 31.1 **Boston Criteria for the Diagnosis of Cerebral Amyloid Angiopathy**

Definite CAA	Confirmation on Postmortem Pathology
Probable CAA with supporting pathology	1. Amyloid deposition in surgical pathology specimen 2. Clinical, radiographic, or pathological history of lobar ICH
Probable CAA without supporting pathology	1. Age older than 55 years 2. Multiple lobar hemorrhages of varying ages/sizes, or single ICH with superficial siderosis 3. Absence of other diagnostic etiologies
Possible CAA	1. Age older than 55 years 2. Clinical or radiographic history of single lobar ICH, or superficial siderosis 3. Absence of other diagnostic etiologies

CAA (Table 31.1). This patient had pathologic confirmation of CAA upon her first presentation, and her subsequent hemorrhages have also all been lobar. She would be classified as having probable CAA with supporting pathology.

This patient had surgical evacuation of her first hemorrhage several years ago. Although this is not standard therapy, the International Surgical Trial in Intracerebral Haemorrhage (STICH) trial showed nonsignificant trend toward benefit in patients who had lobar hemorrhage near the surface. However, the follow-up STICH II trial, which randomized patients with superficial ICH to early surgical evacuation or medical management, found no benefit of surgery on the 6-month rate of death or disability. There was a large degree of crossover (21%) of patients within the medical management group who required surgery for progressive neurological decline despite conservative therapy. Evacuation of clot may be considered in such patients, if it is deemed a life-saving intervention in a patient with a good premorbid baseline. On the other hand, given this patient's diagnosis and severely disabled state, surgery was not considered. There are multiple ongoing clinical trials aimed at assessing the efficacy of minimally invasive surgical methods for the treatment of acute ICH.

Unfortunately, there is no treatment for CAA. Patients are medically managed to lower the risk of recurrent hemorrhage. Due to very high rates of recurrent hemorrhage, anticoagulants are avoided in patients with CAA. The risks and benefits of antiplatelet therapy need to be weighed carefully. Although there are no trials for blood pressure control in patients with CAA, patients with ICH in general have lower recurrence rates with aggressive blood pressure treatment, so this should be instituted in patients with CAA as well. In the Perindopril Protection

Against Recurrent Stroke Study (PROGRESS) trial, patients with active treatment of hypertension were 77% less likely to experience CAA-related ICH.

KEY POINTS TO REMEMBER

· Lobar ICH in an elderly patient may be due to CAA, particularly if the ICH is recurrent and if the patient additionally suffers from dementia.
· Imaging findings of cortical microhemorrhages or superficial siderosis on MRI may support this diagnosis.
· There is no specific medical therapy to prevent hemorrhages in CAA; however, blood pressure should be well controlled and anticoagulation avoided.
· There is no evidence that most patients with acute, superficial ICH respond to surgical evacuation using currently available invasive techniques; however, a subset of patients with good premorbid baseline may be considered for surgery if the hemorrhage is considered life-threatening.

Further Reading

Arima H, Tzourio C, Anderson C, et al.; PROGRESS Collaborative Group. Effects of perindopril-based lowering of blood pressure on intracerebral hemorrhage related to amyloid angiopathy: The PROGRESS trial. *Stroke* 2010;41(2):394–396.

Charidimou A, Martinez-Ramirez S, Shoamanesh A, et al. Cerebral amyloid angiopathy with and without hemorrhage: Evidence for different disease phenotypes. *Neurology* 2015;24;84(12):1206–1212.

Mendelow AD, Gregson BA, Fernandes HM, et al.; STICH investigators. Early surgery versus initial conservative treatment in patients with spontaneous supratentorial intracerebral haematomas in the International Surgical Trial in Intracerebral Haemorrhage (STICH): A randomised trial. *Lancet* 2005;365(9457):387–397.

Mendelow AD, Gregson BA, Rowan EN, et al.; STICH II Investigators. Early surgery versus initial conservative treatment in patients with spontaneous supratentorial lobar intracerebral haematomas (STICH II): A randomised trial. *Lancet* 2013;382(9890):397–408.

Smith EE, Greenberg SM. Clinical diagnosis of cerebral amyloid angiopathy: Validation of the Boston Criteria. *Curr Atheroscler Rep* 2003;5:260–266.

van Etten ES, Auriel E, Haley KE, et al. Incidence of symptomatic hemorrhage in patients with lobar microbleeds. *Stroke* 2014;45(8):2280–2285.

Viswanathan A, Greenberg SM. Cerebral amyloid angiopathy in the elderly. *Ann Neurol* 2011;70:871–880.

32 An Unusual Hemorrhage

A 49-year-old man with no past medical history presented to the ER with vertigo, gait unsteadiness, nausea, and vomiting followed by progressive lethargy. His mental status rapidly declined in the ER, and he was emergently intubated. Initial CT scanning showed hemorrhage in the cerebellum and intraventricular hemorrhage (Figure 32.1). A CTA showed abnormal dilated vessels.

What do you do now?

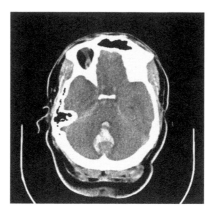

FIGURE 32.1 CT with hemorrhage in the cerebellar vermis and fourth ventricle.

INTRACEREBRAL HEMORRHAGE SECONDARY TO ARTERIOVENOUS MALFORMATION

A young person without a history of hypertension and presenting with a sponta-neous ICH should be evaluated for an underlying lesion. The abnormal vessels on CTA are indicative of arteriovenous malformation (AVM) rupture as an etiol-ogy of this hemorrhage. Arteriovenous malformations are a tangle of vessels with abnormal shunting directly from the arterial to venous system without interven-ing capillaries. AVMs are relatively rare, with a detection rate of approximately 1.2–1.4 per 100,000 persons per year. Some AVMs may remain asymptomatic. Others present with seizure, and approximately half of patients with AVM pres-ent with hemorrhage. Some epidemiological studies suggest a risk of first hem-orrhage of 2–4% per year. Risk factors for hemorrhage include small size, deep drainage, high intranidal pressure, and the presence of feeding artery aneurysm. After a hemorrhage, the risk of rebleeding is elevated and was found in one study to be 18% per year. Although treatment for asymptomatic AVMs is controver-sial, given the high rebleeding rate after a first hemorrhage, the treatment of a ruptured AVM is typically warranted.

The Spetzler–Martin Scale is commonly used to assess surgical risk for treat-ment (Table 32.1). Higher grade lesions are associated with greater morbidity with surgery. This scale was designed to address outcomes with surgery, but it has also been applied to other types of treatment.

Treatment includes surgical resection, embolization in which embolic mate-rial is delivered into feeding arteries, radiosurgery, or a combination of these. There have been no trials to show benefit of any modality over another.

The only randomized trial of the treatment for unruptured AVMs, A Randomized Trial of Unruptured Brain AVMs (ARUBA), studied 223 adults

TABLE 32.1 Spetzler–Martin Scale for the Risk of Surgical Treatment of an AVM

Size	
0–3 cm	1
3.1–6.0 cm	2
>6 cm	3
Location	
Noneloquent	0
Eloquent	1
Deep venous drainage	
Not present	0
Present	1

who underwent interventional therapy (i.e., neurosurgery, embolization, and ste-reotactic radiotherapy, alone or in combination) compared to medical management. This trial was terminated prematurely by the data and safety monitoring board because of the superiority of medical management. The primary outcome of death or symptomatic stroke was reached by 10.1% of the patients in the conservative therapy arm and 30.7% of the patients who underwent intervention. However, this trial is often criticized for not being generalizable to current clinical practice in the United States because there were low rates of AVM treatment with surgical excision (which offers the highest rates of cure).

In this patient, an external ventricular drain was placed for the intraventricular blood. His mental status improved. An angiogram was then done, which

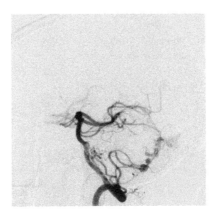

FIGURE 32.2 Cerebral angiogram showing PCA and PICA feeding arteries to the cerebellar AVM.

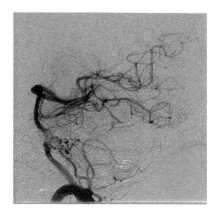

FIGURE 32.3 Cerebral angiogram after embolization and resection.

showed a vermian AVM with a dysplastic aneurysm of posterior inferior cerebellar artery (PICA) (Figure 32.2). This vessel was embolized. The patient then had a suboccipital decompression and AVM resection. Follow-up angiography showed no residual AVM (Figure 32.3). He continued to have residual ataxia.

KEY POINTS TO REMEMBER

· A young patient without hypertension should have an evaluation for underlying cause of ICH.

· AVM is a rare cause of ICH.

· Treatment after hemorrhage may include embolization, surgery, and radiosurgery.

· Most unruptured AVMs may be best managed conservatively.

Further Reading

Mohr JP, Parides MK, Stapf C, et al; for the international ARUBA investigators. Medical management with or without interventional therapy for unruptured brain arteriovenous malformations (ARUBA): A multicentre, non-blinded, randomised trial. *Lancet* 2014;383(9917):614–621.

Ogilvy CS, Stieg PE, Awad I, et al.; Special Writing Group of the Stroke Council, American Stroke Association. AHA Scientific Statement: Recommendations for the management of intracranial arteriovenous malformations: A statement for healthcare professionals from a Special Writing Group of the Stroke Council. *Stroke* 2001;32:1458–1471.

Stapf C, Mast H, Sciacca RR, et al. Predictors of hemorrhage in patients with untreated brain arteriovenous malformation. *Neurology* 2006;66:1350–1355.

van Beijnum J, van der Worp HB, Buis DR, et al. Treatment of brain arteriovenous malformations: A systematic review and meta-analysis. *JAMA* 2011;306:2011–2019.

33 Recurrent Headaches

A 20-year-old college student developed new-onset headache. He had no medical problems. A month prior to presentation, he noticed sharp occipital headaches. They were severe and lasted a few minutes. They occurred five times a day. Over the course of a week, the headaches evolved into a dull constant pain that was relieved with ibuprofen. He eventually had a head CT that showed a hemorrhage. He was neurologically normal and had a normal blood pressure. He then had an MRI (Figure 33.1).

What do I do now?

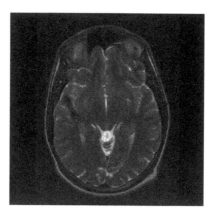

FIGURE 33.1 MRI T2-weighted sequence showing chronic hemosiderin in the right temporal lobe.

INTRACEREBRAL HEMORRHAGE FROM CAVERNOUS MALFORMATION

The lesion in the right temporal lobe of mixed ages of blood is highly suggestive of a cavernous malformation.

Cavernous malformations are circumscribed clusters of dilated, thin-walled capillaries without intervening brain tissue. With the advent of widespread use of MRI, they are being detected more commonly. They are estimated to occur in approximately 1 in 200 people. Approximately 20% of these are familial, with an autosomal dominant mutation in one of three identified genes: *CCM1, CCM2,* and *CCM3*. The remainder are sporadic. The majority of cavernous malformations are supratentorial, and up to one-fourth are associated with developmentally abnormal draining veins. These lesions can cause symptoms of headache and seizure and, depending on location, focal neurological symptoms. Hemorrhage can be devastating and result in severe, progressive neurological deficits. However, given that these lesions are associated with low-flow states, the average hemorrhage rate of unruptured cavernous malformations is less than 1% per year.

Diagnosis is usually by MRI. As in this patient, different ages of blood in a circumscribed lesion can be seen, often in a visual appearance reminiscent of popcorn or a mulberry. Such appearance is produced by the sequential, low-flow oozing of blood from a symptomatic lesion over time. Although MRI is highly sensitive for the detection of these lesions, cavernous malformations do not appear on conventional angiography. In some cases, however, an angiogram may be done to exclude an arteriovenous malformation.

When should such lesions be treated? This is a controversial area, and there are no randomized trials to guide management. To approach this rationally, one must understand the natural history and risk of hemorrhage before considering treatment.

Unfortunately, results of studies that have evaluated risk of hemorrhage from cavernous malformations are mixed because of heterogeneity in the study methodologies. The risks appear to range between 0.25% and 4.5% per year for recurrent hemorrhage. Lesion location also seems to be important, with deep or infratentorial lesions more likely to bleed. The presence of multiple lesions or cavernous malformations associated with developmental venous anomalies also may have higher bleeding risk.

In the largest prospective study on the subject, investigators followed 292 patients with known cavernous malformation to determine risk factors and rates of hemorrhage. In this study, patients who initially presented with a hemorrhage had a 6% annual rate of hemorrhage compared with 0.33% in patients whose cavernous malformation was detected incidentally. The median time to second hemorrhage was 8 months, and the risk declined after the first 2 years. In this series, 80% of patients who presented with hemorrhage had no recurrent hemorrhage for 10 years.

Surgical intervention is considered when there is progressive neurological deficit due to recurrent hemorrhage or intractable epilepsy. In deep and eloquent regions, the risk of hemorrhage needs to be weighed against the morbidity associated with microsurgery, which may be as high as 10% depending on the lesion location. Stereotactic radiosurgery has also been used in patients with surgically inaccessible lesions. The efficacy of this intervention in reducing hemorrhage rates is not well defined, and there is evidence that radiosurgery may lead to worsened neurological deficits with time compared to the natural history of cavernous malformations.

Recently, a prospective, nonrandomized trial was published regarding the treatment of cavernous malformations in 134 adult Scottish patients. The authors compared medical management to intervention with either microsurgical excision or stereotactic radiosurgery, which was left to the treating physician's discretion. However, only 19% of the patients were treated with microsurgery (none received radiosurgery). Those who underwent surgical intervention were younger and more likely to present with ICH, neurological deficits, or seizures. Patients who were treated conservatively were more than twice as likely to have excellent disability outcomes and more than three times less likely to have the secondary outcome of ICH or focal neurological deficit on 5-year follow-up. Nearly all of the hemorrhage events or neurological deficits occurred within 30 days of surgery. Mortality was similar (12%) between the medical and surgical groups. The annual hemorrhage rate for all-comers in this cohort was 3.73%. This trial has cast further skepticism on the utility of surgical intervention for cavernous malformations using currently available techniques. Nevertheless, a randomized trial is needed to further assess the risks and benefits of surgical excision for cavernous malformations.

This patient had an angiogram that revealed no underlying AVM. He had evidence of a developmental venous anomaly, which is often seen in association with cavernous malformations. Because he had no neurological symptoms despite evidence of hemorrhage, he was managed conservatively. He understood the risk of possible seizure and hemorrhage. He was monitored for clinical symptoms, and he remained symptom-free for the entire 8 years of follow-up.

KEY POINTS TO REMEMBER

- Cavernous malformations may cause symptoms due to recurrent bleeding or seizures.
- Intervention should be considered in patients with progressive neurological symptoms or refractory epilepsy. However, current nonrandomized data suggest that nonsurgical treatment of these lesions may be superior.
- Cavernous malformations may be familial.

Further Reading

Batra S, Rigamonti K, Rigamonti D. Management of hemorrhage from cavernous malformations. *Curr Atheroscler Rep* 2012;14:360–365.

Del Curling OJr, Kelly DLJr, Elster AD, et al. An analysis of the natural history of cavernous angiomas. *J Neurosurg* 1991;75:702–708.

Flemming KD, Link MJ, Christianson TJ, et al. Prospective hemorrhage risk of intracerebral cavernous malformations. *Neurology* 2012;78:632–636.

Moultrie F, Horne MA, Josephson CB, et al; on behalf of the Scottish Audit of Intracranial Vascular Malformations (SAIVMs). Outcome after surgical or conservative management of cerebral cavernous malformations. *Neurology* 2014;83(7):582–589.

34 Progressive Gait Dysfunction

A 79-year-old man with a history of treated renal cell carcinoma developed progressive gait difficulty. He first noticed some mild symptoms of imbalance 2 years ago. During the past several months, he has had more difficulty walking. He has also noticed decreased sensation in the legs and urinary urgency. He had no back pain or prior trauma. His strength was normal on examination, but he had impaired sensation in the legs. He had spine imaging that revealed vascular flow voids along the dorsal aspect of the thoracic spine (Figure 34.1).

What do you do now?

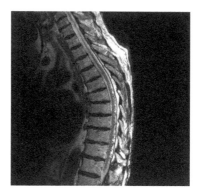

FIGURE 34.1 MRI showing vascular flow voids along the dorsal aspect of the thoracic spine suggestive of a dural AVF.

DURAL ARTERIOVENOUS FISTULA OF THE SPINE

The clinical symptoms of a gradually progressive gait disorder with sensory change and urinary dysfunction should raise the suspicion for a spinal cord disorder. MRI is an appropriate imaging modality to detect lesions in the spinal cord. Vascular causes of myelopathy are rare but should be considered. In this case, the abnormal flow voids along the spinal cord are dilated veins, suggesting increased venous congestion as seen in dural arteriovenous fistulas (AVFs). If flow voids are not apparent, contrast MRI may also show enhancing dilated vessels. Spinal angiography is the definitive test to confirm the diagnosis. Although spinal vascular malformations are rare, dural AVFs account for the majority of vascular lesions within the spine. Unlike spinal arteriovenous malformations, which cause abrupt neurological change as a result of hemorrhage, spinal dural AVFs tend to result in a progressive myelopathy through venous congestion and cord edema.

A dural AVF is an abnormal communication between an artery and vein of the dura, a covering surrounding the spinal cord. The fistula is formed by a radicular artery that feeds directly into a medullary vein. This causes venous congestion as the arterial blood is shunted into the venous system, resulting in dilation of the venous plexus along the spinal cord. Spinal cord symptoms develop due to increasing vascular congestion of the cord. Sluggish venous drainage of the cord leads to progressive myelopathic symptoms, which may include extremity weakness, changes in tone, gait instability, numbness, and urinary or sexual dysfunction. MRI can show edema within the spinal cord.

The pathophysiology of these acquired lesions is unknown. However, similar to brain dural AVFs, chronic venous thrombosis and trauma may predispose to

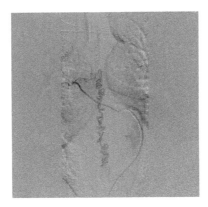

FIGURE 34.2 Spinal angiogram demonstrating the dural AVF.

fistula formation. The typical onset of symptoms is in the fifth or sixth decade, and men are more commonly affected than women. The thoracic cord is the most common site of fistula formation.

Treatment can be endovascular, surgical, or a combination of these two approaches. With endovascular therapy, the feeding artery is identified by angiography and embolized with material to occlude the artery. Embolization of the fistula is less invasive, but there is potential for infarction of the cord. Surgical treatment requires identification of the fistula and surgical obliteration. In one large series of treated patients with spinal dural AVFs, endovascular therapy was successful in 77% of patients and surgical obliteration was used in those with residual shunt. Patients in this series had good recovery of neurologic function, with more than 70% having improved gait and leg sensation and 50% having improved micturition.

This patient had an angiogram that confirmed the diagnosis. Segmental arterial injections showed a T7 feeding artery with early venous drainage and dilated perimedullary veins (Figure 34.2). He was unable to have direct embolization of the T7 feeding artery due to tortuosity. He had surgical laminectomy and obliteration of the fistula. Follow-up angiography showed no residual shunting.

KEY POINTS TO REMEMBER

· Dural AVFs are a rare cause of progressive myelopathic symptoms due to venous congestion and resultant spinal cord edema.
· Treatment is with embolization or surgical obliteration of the fistula.
· Symptoms may be reversible if treated early.

Further Reading

Kirsh M, Berg-Dammer E, Musahl C, et al. Endovascular management of spinal dural arteriovenous fistulas in 78 patients. *Neuroradiology* 2013;55:337–343.

Marcus J, Schwarz J, Singh IP, et al. Spinal dural arteriovenous fistulas: A review. *Curr Atheroscler Rep* 2013;15:335.

35 Worst Headache of Her Life

A 43-year-old woman with a history of tobacco abuse and
hypertension controlled with medications presented to the
ER with sudden-onset severe throbbing, global, persistent
headache followed by syncope. On evaluation in the
ER, her vitals were normal, and she was neurologically
intact without signs of meningismus or focal neurological
deficits. Initial CT scan was interpreted as normal
(Figure 35.1).

What do you do now?

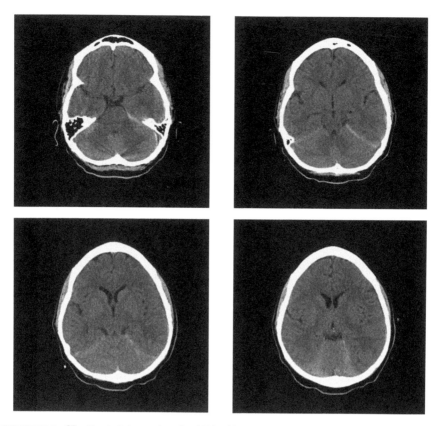

FIGURE 35.1 CT without obvious subarachnoid blood but hyperdensity along the tentorium.

ANEURYSMAL SUBARACHNOID HEMORRHAGE

Acute worst headache of life requires immediate evaluation for aneurysmal SAH. The incidence of SAH is 2–16 per 100,000. Although not a common diagnosis, SAH should never be missed because the mortality is very high (up to 50%). The risk of aneurysmal rebleeding after the initial hemorrhage is also high (15–20% within the first 2 weeks), and recurrent hemorrhage leads to further increases in mortality. In addition, the morbidity can be substantial; many patients are left with permanent cognitive deficits impairing functional status and quality of life.

CT scan done acutely has more than a 95% sensitivity for detecting subarachnoid blood. The location of blood on imaging can indicate the location of ruptured aneurysm. For example, MCA aneurysms may have focal clot within the Sylvian fissure. ACA aneurysms may have more blood within the interhemispheric fissure. Often, blood is distributed throughout the suprasellar cistern and cannot provide a clue to aneurysm location. In this patient, the subarachnoid

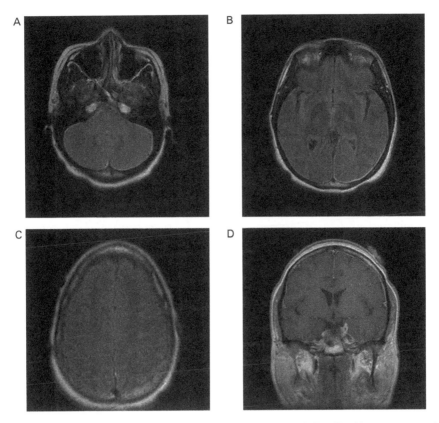

FIGURE 35.2   (A–C) FLAIR with subtle subarachnoid and subdural blood. (D) MRI with contrast, coronal view showing left posterior communicating artery aneurysm.

component of the hemorrhage was not obvious on CT. The hemorrhage in this case is more subdural and can be seen along the tentorium.

It is important to note that the sensitivity of a CT scan for SAH decreases continuously with time as the blood products are degraded, and rates of detection can be as low as 50% by 1 week. Therefore, clinical suspicion for SAH with a negative head CT requires a lumbar puncture to evaluate for xanthochromia. Xanthochromia should be present for up to 2 weeks post-hemorrhage and would confirm a diagnosis of SAH. MRI technology may also be able to pick up subtle abnormalities in the cerebral sulci, consistent with subarachnoid blood, when CT fails to do so (Figure 35.2). In this patient, an MRI was immediately done, which showed subdural and subarachnoid hemorrhage as well as the location of the aneurysm in the posterior communicating artery (P Comm).

The severity of clinical presentation has been found to be the strongest predictor of clinical outcome. The Hunt–Hess grading system is a commonly used tool to quantify a patient's deficit. This score also has prognostic implications, with higher scores associated with worse outcomes (Box 35.1).

Our patient had a Hunt–Hess grade 1, suggesting a good prognosis. Conversely, patients with poor-grade SAH (Hunt–Hess 4 or 5) have a mortality >70%. In modern times, these mortality rates have been decreasing due to improved management of patients in dedicated neurological ICUs and the advent of endovascular coiling techniques to treat ruptured aneurysms.

Once the diagnosis is made, patients should be monitored closely in an ICU, preferably one dedicated to the neurosciences. This allows for frequent neurological exams, hemodynamic monitoring, and management by a team familiar with SAH treatment. Because of the risk of rebleeding, the aneurysm should be treated as quickly as possible. While awaiting treatment, blood pressure should be monitored closely and treated to keep the SBP <160 to lower the risk of rebleeding. However, care should be taken not to lower the blood pressure so much as to compromise cerebral perfusion in patients with elevated ICP. In patients with elevated ICP or hydrocephalus, prompt neurosurgical evaluation is required for placement of an external ventriculostomy drain. If the aneurysm cannot be treated quickly, short-term use of antifibrinolytic therapy (e.g., aminocaproic acid) can be initiated to help prevent rebleeding.

Treatment is either surgical clipping of the aneurysm or endovascular coiling. Choice of treatment strategy depends on the anatomy of the aneurysm (location, size, and aneurysm neck size) and the patient's risk factors. In general, endovascular treatment seems to have lower morbidity and mortality. The largest randomized trial comparing coiling to clipping in patients whose aneurysm was amenable to either form of treatment is the International Subarachnoid Aneurysm Trial (ISAT). ISAT demonstrated that despite a higher risk of rebleeding with coil embolization, coiling was associated with higher rates of independent survival over at least 10 years of follow-up.

After treatment, there is risk of vasospasm and delayed cerebral ischemia. Subarachnoid blood can cause local vessel irritation, causing spasm. This can lead to stroke, resulting in increased rates of morbidity and mortality. Vasospasm usually peaks 5–10 days after a hemorrhage, but it can be observed from 3 to 21 days post-SAH. Serial transcranial Dopplers are often used to screen for increasing velocities, which may suggest developing spasm. Ultrasound technology allows for bedside assessment and carries less risk than repeating either CT or conventional angiography. Patients are typically treated prophylactically with a calcium channel blocker, nimodipine, and hydration to maintain euvolemia. If symptomatic vasospasm develops, hypertensive therapy or angioplasty, with or without intra-arterial infusion of calcium channel blockers, may be considered.

Other medical complications are common following SAH. Fluid and electrolyte imbalances are frequently encountered. Hyponatremia may develop from varying mechanisms, including cerebral salt wasting syndrome and the syndrome of inappropriate antidiuretic hormone secretion (SIADH). This is an important clinical distinction to make, given that aggressive volume resuscitation would combat cerebral salt wasting and fluid restriction the other. Fever of central (noninfectious) origin could represent a marker of a systemic inflammatory state in response to hemorrhage, and maintenance of normothermia may improve outcomes. Up to one-fourth of patients experience seizures. Although routine prophylaxis against seizures is not recommended, short-term antiepileptic therapy is reasonable in the immediate post-hemorrhagic period. This is particularly important for those patients with unprotected aneurysms, in whom a seizure could theoretically result in re-rupture. Cardiac injury can also be noted in response to SAH and should be evaluated if clinically suspected.

In this patient, an angiogram confirmed the presence of a bilobed posterior communicating artery aneurysm with a narrow neck projecting posterolaterally

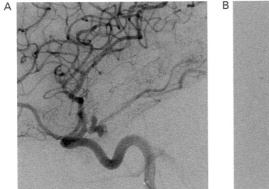 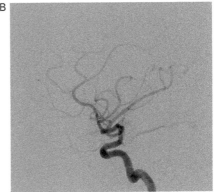

FIGURE 35.3 (A) Cerebral angiogram showing bilobed P Comm aneurysm. (B) Cerebral angiogram post-coiling of aneurysm.

(Figure 35.3). Coil embolization of the aneurysm was done without complications. The patient had an uneventful course in the neurological ICU and did not develop any symptomatic vasospasm. She made a complete recovery and was discharged home with no neurological symptoms. Follow-up angiograms done at 6 months and at 1 year showed no evidence of recurrence or recanalization of the aneurysm.

KEY POINTS TO REMEMBER

- Sudden, severe headache requires rapid evaluation for SAH.
- A negative CT with high clinical suspicion for SAH warrants a lumbar puncture to assess for xanthochromia.
- Morbidity and mortality are high from aneurysmal SAH so treatment needs to be initiated quickly.
- In patients with aneurysms amenable to both surgical clipping and endovascular coiling, coiling results in higher rates of independent survival despite a higher risk of rebleeding.
- Nimodipine has been shown to improve outcomes and prevent cerebral ischemia in patients at risk for vasospasm.
- Vasospasm should be closely monitored for, and if found, treatment options include hydration, induced hypertension, angioplasty, and intra-arterial infusion of vasodilators.

Further Reading

Connolly ES, Rabinstein AA, Carhuapoma JR, et al. Guidelines for the management of aneurysmal subarachnoid hemorrhage: A guideline for healthcare professionals from the American Heart Association/American Stroke Association. *Stroke* 2012;43:1711–1737.

Hunt WE, Hess RM. Surgical risk as related to time of intervention in the repair of intracranial aneurysms. *J Neurosurg* 1968;28:14.

Molyneux AJ, Birks J, Clarke A, et al. The durability of endovascular coiling versus neurosurgical clipping of ruptured cerebral aneurysms: 18 year follow-up of the UK cohort of the International Subarachnoid Aneurysm Trial (ISAT). *Lancet* 2015:385:691–697.

36 An Incidental Finding

A 41-year-old man with a history of high cholesterol and active tobacco abuse was well until 2 months ago. He noted a gradual onset of right-sided headache. He described the headache as pressure. He had no nausea or vomiting but did report bilateral blurred vision and photophobia. The headache is daily and constant, but he has relief with ibuprofen. He has had no motor, sensory, or language symptoms. His neurological examination is normal. He had an MRI and MRA of the brain to evaluate this new-onset headache. Imaging revealed a 5-mm aneurysm of the right internal carotid artery siphon.

What do you do now?

ASYMPTOMATIC INTRACRANIAL ANEURYSM

With the widespread use of brain imaging such as MRI and MRA for symptoms such as headache, we are incidentally detecting more intracranial aneurysms. The knowledge that there is 50% mortality with rupture of an aneurysm provokes much anxiety. Patients naturally want to know their risk of bleeding and the potential treatments to prevent aneurysmal rupture. How to address an asymptomatic aneurysm is a commonly encountered clinical question. The prevalence of intracranial aneurysms is estimated at 2% or 3% of the general population, and it may be higher in women, older patients, and people of Asian or Finnish ancestry. Despite their frequent identification, routine screening for unruptured intracranial aneurysms is typically not recommended unless a patient has two or more first-degree relatives with aneurysms or a genetic condition (e.g., autosomal dominant polycystic kidney disease) that predisposes to aneurysm formation.

In order to decide on the treatment for an incidentally discovered intracranial aneurysm, it is essential to evaluate the risk of bleeding (based on the suspected natural history of the aneurysm) weighed against the risks and benefits of the proposed treatment method. Multiple factors play a role in the risk of hemorrhage from an unruptured intracranial aneurysm and should be considered in decisions to manage an aneurysm either expectantly or surgically. Risk factors linked to aneurysmal rupture include cigarette smoking, hypertension, aneurysm growth and morphology, younger age, female sex, and prior personal or family history of SAH. However, the location and size of an aneurysm have consistently been recognized as crucial determinants to its risk of bleeding. Still much is uncertain regarding the natural history of asymptomatic aneurysms, and there remains disagreement regarding which patient and aneurysm characteristics are most important when deciding on intervention. Regardless of the chosen treatment strategy, it is typically recommended to institute blood pressure management and tobacco cessation, although there is no direct, prospective evidence demonstrating that control of these modifiable risk factors reduces rates of aneurysmal SAH.

When deciding if an incidental aneurysm should be referred for a surgical or endovascular procedure, a clinician should consider both the size and the location of the aneurysm. The first question is whether the aneurysm is intradural or extradural. Cavernous carotid aneurysms are extradural and hence do not cause SAH when they rupture. However, such aneurysms can cause symptoms due to compression of other structures. For example, eye movement abnormalities can be seen due to compression of the third, fourth, and sixth cranial nerves. Treatment of cavernous carotid aneurysms is usually warranted only if they cause compressive symptoms. Carotid aneurysms that are intradural cause SAH and therefore may be considered for intervention depending on other patient and aneurysm characteristics.

The next level of determining bleeding risk is whether the aneurysm is within the anterior or posterior circulation. Then the size should be considered. There exist two large, prospective studies that evaluate the bleeding risk of unruptured intracranial aneurysms, primarily based on the size and location of the aneurysm. The International Study of Unruptured Intracranial Aneurysms (ISUIA) study found that in patients without history of prior ruptured aneurysm, the cumulative risk of SAH in 5 years was dependent on both location and size (Table 36.1).

A Japanese study showed that anterior and posterior communicating artery aneurysms were more likely to rupture compared to other locations. This study also found morphology of the aneurysm to be important. Aneurysms with a daughter sac (an irregular protrusion of the aneurysm wall) were also more likely to rupture. However, decisions on asymptomatic aneurysm management are rather complex, involving multiple clinical factors, and may be best judged by a multidisciplinary assessment of treatment risks and benefits.

When referring a patient for intervention, the estimated risk of future hemorrhage is weighed against the procedural risks. This requires the balancing of an immediate operative risk with a delayed, potential bleeding risk and therefore should include a careful discussion with the patient and consideration of his or her preferences. The two options for treatment are surgical aneurysm clipping and endovascular coiling. In the United States, coiling has surpassed clipping as the most common method of treatment. Although there are no randomized trials comparing these two techniques for unruptured aneurysms, several retrospective analyses have been performed on large national databases demonstrating the improved procedural morbidity and mortality observed with modern coiling techniques. In one such study of the Nationwide Inpatient Sample, poor outcome (defined as discharge to long-term facility) was seen in 14% of 29,918 patients treated surgically versus 5% of 34,125 patients treated endovascularly. In-hospital mortality was also significantly higher with surgery. In addition, several studies, including the ISUIA, suggest that patients older than age 50 years

TABLE 36.1 **Size of Aneurysm**

	Size			
Location	<7 mm	7–12 mm	13–24 mm	>25 mm
Anterior (%)	0	2.6	14.5	40
Posterior (%)	2.5	14.5	18.4	50

may benefit from coiling of unruptured aneurysms. Data from randomized trials evaluating the treatment of ruptured aneurysms must be considered with caution in populations with unruptured aneurysms. Nevertheless, note that in the ISAT trial, which compared clipping and coiling in patients who suffered SAH, those who were treated with surgery had higher morbidity and mortality despite a higher rate of successful treatment and lower long-term risk of rebleeding. Overall, it appears that endovascular treatment is associated with better outcomes, but future randomized trials in unruptured aneurysms are needed.

For this patient, the distinction of intra- versus extradural location of the aneurysm was not clear on noninvasive imaging. Sizing is also more accurate on a conventional angiogram. For these reasons, this patient had an angiogram to determine the exact location. He was found to have a 3.4-mm intradural hypophyseal aneurysm.

The small size in a favorable location is associated with low risk of hemorrhage. He was counseled to stop smoking because this is a risk factor for hemorrhage. He was also advised to monitor his blood pressure and ensure that it is treated if necessary. He had a follow-up MRA at 1 year, and no enlargement was detected. He remained symptom free.

KEY POINTS TO REMEMBER

- Routine screening for intracranial aneurysms should only be performed in patients with two or more relatives with aneurysms or a predisposing genetic condition.
- Symptomatic, large, and/or growing aneurysms should be considered for treatment, particularly if they are in a high-risk location.
- Asymptomatic aneurysms in a patient who had prior SAH, or a family history, should be considered for treatment because risk of hemorrhage is higher.
- Small aneurysms may be monitored.
- Treatment needs to be individualized. Surgery has been associated with neurological disability and cognitive impairment. Endovascular coiling may be associated with a higher rate of incomplete obliteration. There are no randomized trial data in patients with unruptured aneurysms.
- Modifiable risk factors associated with aneurysm growth and rupture (hypertension and tobacco use) should be addressed.

Further Reading

Brinjikji W, Rabinstein AA, Nasr DM, et al. Better outcomes with treatment by coiling relative to clipping of unruptured intracranial aneurysms in the United States, 2001–2008. *Am J Neuroradiol* 2011;32(6):1071–1075.

Etminan N, Beseoglu K, Barrow DL, et al. Multidisciplinary consensus on assessment of unruptured intracranial aneurysms: Proposal of an international research group. *Stroke* 2014;45:1523–1530.

International Study of Unruptured Intracranial Aneurysms Investigators. Unruptured intracranial aneurysms: Natural history, clinical outcome, and risks of surgical and endovascular treatment. *Lancet* 2003;362:103–110.

Thompson BG, Brown RD, Sepideh AH, et al. Guidelines for the management of patients with unruptured intracranial aneurysms: A guidelines for healthcare professionals from the American Heart Association/American Stroke Association. *Stroke* 2015;46(8):2368–2400.

The UCAS Japan Investigators. The natural course of unruptured cerebral aneurysms in a Japanese cohort. *N Engl J Med* 2012;366:2474–2482.

37 Forget About It

A 69-year-old woman with mechanical aortic valve replacement, coronary artery disease, and hypertension comes to the office for evaluation of memory change. Her husband notes that he came home one day and she could not remember what happened that day. It was a sudden change. Since then, she has had difficulty with short-term memory. She forgets what she said, what plans she made for dinner, and where things are located. She needs to write everything down so she does not forget. She does not get lost, but her husband accompanies her everywhere. Her husband has started paying the bills and managing the finances.

On examination, she did not know the date. She had difficulty with complex commands and calculations. She had difficulty with short-term recall. The rest of her exam was normal. Her MRI done several weeks after onset of symptoms showed chronic infarcts (Figure 37.1).

What do you do now?

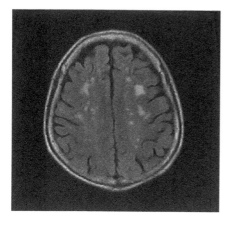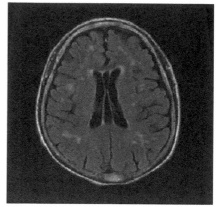

FIGURE 37.1 MRI of the brain showing scattered, mostly subcortical, old cerebral infarcts in the bilateral hemispheres.

VASCULAR DEMENTIA

The evaluation of a patient with cognitive complaints includes brain imaging. In this patient, evidence of multiple chronic bilateral infarcts and abrupt onset of symptoms raise the concern for vascular dementia.

Vascular dementia is a complicated diagnosis to make because there are no broadly accepted clinical criteria for the disorder. Dementia, historically, has required memory impairment. However, vascular disease may cause cognitive impairment in other domains without memory impairment.

The National Institute of Neurological Disorders and Stroke (NINDS) and the Association Internationale pour la Recherché et l'Enseignement en Neurosciences (AIREN) created the NINDS–AIREN criteria for vascular dementia. They require all of the following for a diagnosis of probable vascular dementia:

1. Cognitive decline (which impairs activities of daily living) in memory and two or more other domains (orientation, attention, language, visuospatial function, motor control, and praxis).
2. Cerebrovascular disease with findings on exam consistent with stroke, and imaging findings of multiple large vessel infarcts, multiple subcortical lacunes, extensive periventricular white matter disease, or a strategically placed single infarct (within an area that typically subserves cognitive domains, such as the thalamus, basal forebrain, or the PCA or ACA territory).
3. Onset of dementia occurred within 3 months after a stroke, with an abrupt deterioration, or stepwise progression.

Formal neuropsychological testing is preferred to determine the cognitive domains affected and severity of deficit. However, simple bedside screening tools have been developed to quickly assess patients. One such test is the Montreal Cognitive Assessment (MoCA) (Figure 37.2). This assessment scale

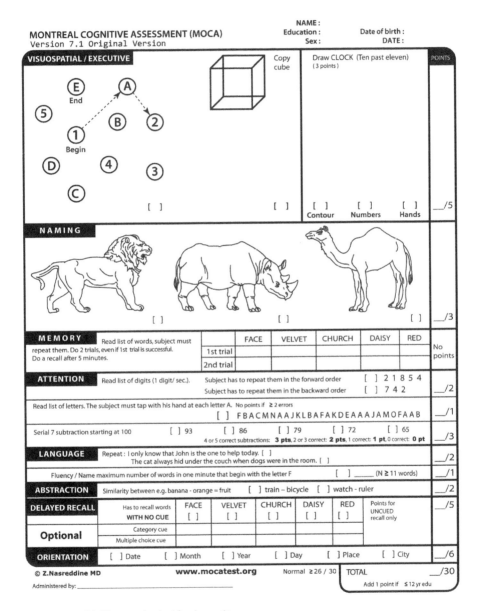

FIGURE 37.2 MoCA screening tool for dementia.

Source: Copyright Z. Nasreddine, MD. Reproduced with permission. Copies are available at http://www.mocatest.org.

may be more sensitive to detecting abnormalities of attention and executive function, which are more commonly seen in vascular dementia than in Alzheimer's disease.

Vascular dementia is a heterogeneous group of disorders. Multiple cortical strokes, a single strategic stroke, multiple subcortical strokes, and chronic white matter disease have all been associated with cognitive decline and have very different clinical presentations and likely different pathophysiology of dementia. Furthermore, recall bias may occur in which family members report acute onset of symptoms after an event such as head trauma or stroke, but there may have been chronic decline prior to that which was due to Alzheimer's disease. This makes treatment trials difficult because the treatment group is heterogeneous.

Drugs used in Alzheimer's disease have been tested in vascular dementia, and results have been mixed. Trials of donepezil have shown some benefit. In one randomized trial of donepezil in 616 patients, greater improvement in cognitive function was seen in patients on donepezil compared with placebo. Improvement was also seen in global function. Cholinesterase inhibitors and memantine may have a small benefit in cognition, but data are conflicting and benefit is significantly less than that seen in Alzheimer's disease.

This patient had sudden onset of symptoms, a significant vascular disease history, and MRI findings supporting a diagnosis of vascular dementia. She had cognitive decline in more than one domain and was requiring more help with daily activities. She was diagnosed with vascular dementia. She was placed on a medical regimen to lower the risk of recurrent stroke that included continuing anticoagulation for her mechanical heart valve. She had aggressive treatment of her hypertension and was monitored for dyslipidemia and diabetes.

She was also placed on donepezil and memantine for the possibility of mixed dementia with vascular and Alzheimer's features.

KEY POINTS TO REMEMBER

- Cognitive impairment is common following stroke, but it may be heterogeneous in presentation.
- Given the heterogeneity of vascular dementia and the overlap of Alzheimer's and vascular dementia, standardized diagnostic criteria (NINDS–AIREN) for vascular dementia have been proposed.
- Acetylcholinesterase inhibitors and memantine may be used off-label to treat vascular dementia patients.

Further Reading

O'Brien JT, Thomas A. Vascular dementia. *Lancet* 2015;386:1698–1706.

Roman GC, Tatemichi TK, Erkinjuntti T, et al. Vascular dementia: Diagnostic criteria for research studies: Report of the NINDS-AIREN International Workshop. *Neurology* 1993;43(2):250–260.

Wilkinson D, Boody R, Helme R, et al. Donepezil in vascular dementia. *Neurology* 2003;61:479–486.

38 Seizures, Sadness, and Spasticity

A 67-year-old woman with atrial fibrillation and recent stroke comes to the ER with a new-onset seizure. The seizure was described as a 3-minute episode in which her left arm started to uncontrollably shake. She then fell to the ground with brief generalized shaking. On evaluation, the patient is now alert, appropriate, and oriented, with a spastic weakness of her left arm and minor left facial droop. The patient suffered an embolic stroke of the right MCA territory 6 months prior, which has left her with a residual hemiparesis. Unfortunately, she has been lost to follow-up and has not seen a doctor or participated in a rehabilitation program. She has developed pain and stiffness of her left arm, which is held in a flexed position. When talking with the patient about her recent stroke, she becomes tearful and endorses a depressed mood and frustration regarding her new disability. She asks if there is anything you can do to help improve her stroke recovery.

What do you do now?

POST-STROKE REHABILITATION

Stroke affects 800,000 people annually in the United States and is a leading cause of serious long-term disability. A total of 40% of stroke patients are left with some form of moderate to severe disability. After discharge, patients with stroke are at risk for multiple medical and neurological complications that could result in further morbidity and loss of quality of life. It is imperative to recognize the myriad of potential neurological issues a patient with stroke may face and to appropriately address them as they arise in order to reduce disability and optimize a patient's recovery (Box 38.1). Effective rehabilitation, in particular, can enhance the recovery process and minimize functional disability. If undergoing a therapeutic rehabilitation program, patients may expect to clinically improve for up to 6 or more months following stroke.

Although the exact timing, intensity, and duration of physical therapy have not been precisely defined, typical guideline recommendations are to initiate rehabilitation therapy early, once medical stability is reached and after the patient exits the hyperacute phase of stroke. Patients should continue with dedicated speech, occupational, and physical therapy as needed in order to adapt, strengthen, and provide the best chance to reestablish a premorbid level of functional independence. Rehabilitation efforts should be multidisciplinary and organized, an approach that has been found to significantly reduce death or dependency if initiated within 1 week of stroke. However, very early, intensive rehabilitation therapy within 24 hours of stroke was shown to result in higher rates of 3-month disability in A Very Early Rehabilitation Trial for Stroke (AVERT), a recent randomized trial of 2104 stroke patients.

Unfortunately, this patient has ignored advice to participate in a rehabilitation program and is left with significant weakness and spasticity post-stroke. Spasticity following muscle paresis is very common following stroke and can

---

BOX 38.1 **Post-Stroke Neurologic and Neuropsychiatric Complications**

Spasticity
Dementia and other cognitive disturbances
Seizures
Falls and gait disturbance
Depression and other mood disturbances
Dysphagia, leading to aspiration
Immobility, leading to venous thromboembolism
Syndromes of apathy, amotivation, abulia, and neglect
Inability to communicate, aphasia
Neurogenic incontinence

be seen in 40% or more of stroke patients. Muscle spasticity can lead to discomfort and further reduced mobility beyond what is observed with the initial degree of weakness. Systemic medications acting on the gamma-aminobutyric acid system are commonly used oral antispasmodics. These include baclofen, benzodiazepines, and gabapentin or pregabalin. The use of these medications is often limited by various potential side effects, including muscle weakness, sedation, dizziness, and hypotension. Other medications are used with success in certain patients experiencing spasticity (Box 38.2). There are surgical options as well, such as tendon and soft tissue release or the use of an intrathecal baclofen pump; however, these are usually reserved for patients with more severe spasticity. Botulinum toxin type A is the gold standard treatment for patients with focal spasticity. If a patient is noted to have focal spasticity and is not responding to, or is unable to tolerate, oral antispasmodics, he or she should be referred to a clinician who can perform botulinum toxin injections. Multiple randomized studies confirm the long-term, yet reversible, benefit of botulinum toxin on muscle tone and functionality. Nevertheless, none of these treatments should preclude efforts to prevent spasticity by employing adequate physical therapy exercises and passive stretching in patients with motor paresis.

Seizures are a well-known consequence of stroke, which accounts for more than 30% of newly diagnosed seizures in older populations. Current guidelines do not recommend seizure prophylaxis for patients with stroke. However, if a patient develops recurrent seizures, treatment with antiepileptic medications is indicated. When selecting antiepileptic drugs, it is important to note that commonly prescribed seizure medications such as phenytoin, phenobarbital,

---

BOX 38.2 **Potential Treatments for Spasticity**

Physical therapy
    Passive stretching and muscular strengthening
    Neuromuscular electrical stimulation
Oral antispasmodics
    Baclofen, benzodiazepines, gabapentin, pregabalin
    Tizanidine, dantrolene
    Cannabinoids
Intrathecal baclofen or phenol
Botulinum toxin injection
Phenol nerve block
Orthopedic surgery
    Tendon and soft tissue release
Neurosurgery
    Dorsal rhizotomy

carbamazepine, and valproic acid may interact with warfarin and require dosage adjustments, if being used for secondary stroke prevention. Given that many patients with stroke are older in age, clinicians must consider, for example, relative dosage lowering to account for the effect that aging has on pharmacokinetics and pharmacodynamics, as well as the medication's effect on bone density for agents such as phenytoin, phenobarbital, and valproic acid. Levetiracetem and lamotrigine may have the best tolerability in this age group.

Post-stroke depression is highly prevalent (seen in at least 30% of patients) and should be screened for in patients with stroke. Depressed mood may impair active patient participation in the rehabilitation process. There is evidence that treatment of depression with serotonergic modulators may improve motor function following stroke. In a randomized controlled trial of 118 adult stroke patients with hemiparesis who were treated with 20 mg of fluoxetine or placebo, those treated with fluoxetine scored higher on a commonly used motor scale 3 months after their index stroke. This suggests the possibility that exogenous serotonin may modulate brain plasticity in the recovery process. Patients who display a significant component of apathy may respond to stimulant medications or dopamine agonists.

This patient was discharged on a selective serotonin reuptake inhibitor (escitalopram) and was started on a titration of lamotrigine to treat her seizure disorder. Secondarily, lamotrigine may have the additional benefit of mood stabilization in this patient. She was started on an outpatient physical therapy and occupational therapy program and was referred to a specialist who started botulinum toxin injections for her left arm spasticity.

KEY POINTS TO REMEMBER

· A multidisciplinary, organized rehabilitation program—including physical, speech, and occupational therapy—is integral to restoring function and preventing complications post-stroke.
· Although oral antispasmodics are beneficial for patients with generalized spasticity, they are often not tolerated at high doses. Botulinum toxin injections are useful for focal spasticity. Refractory spasticity may be treated with surgical options.
· Seizures are relatively common post-stroke, and drug interactions and patient side effects need to be considered when selecting an antiepileptic medication.
· Depression is very common post-stroke and may impair rehabilitation efforts. Selective serotonin reuptake inhibitors may improve motor outcomes post-stroke.

Further Reading

Bernhardt J, Langhorne P, et al.; AVERT Trial Collaboration Group. Efficacy and safety of very early mobilisation within 24 h of stroke onset (AVERT): A randomised controlled trial. *Lancet* 2015;386(9988):46–55.

Chollet F, Tardy J, Albucher JF, et al. Fluoxetine for motor recovery after acute ischaemic stroke (FLAME): A randomised placebo-controlled trial. *Lancet Neurol* 2011;10(2):123–130.

Duncan PW, Zorowitz R, Bates B, et al. Management of adult stroke rehabilitation care: A clinical practice guideline. *Stroke* 2005;36:e100–e143.

Ferlazzo E, Sueri C, Gasparini S, et al. Challenges in the pharmacological management of epilepsy and its causes in the elderly. *Pharmacol Res*. 2016;106:21–26.

Kaňovský P, Slawek J, Denes Z, et al. Efficacy and safety of treatment with incobotulinum toxin A (botulinum neurotoxin type A free from complexing proteins; NT 201) in post-stroke upper limb spasticity. *J Rehabil Med* 2011;43(6):486–492.

Index

Page numbers followed by *f* indicate figures and those followed by *t* indicate tables.

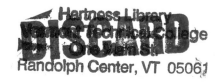